DASH Diet Cookbook For Women

Simple Dr. Cole's Meal Plan | Delicious and Affordable Low Sodium Recipes to Weight Loss and Lower Blood Pressure

By Janeth Cole

The content contained within this book may not be reproduced, duplicated or transmitted without direct written permission from the author or the publisher. Under no circumstances will any blame or legal responsibility be held against the publisher, or author, for any damages, reparation, or monetary loss due to the information contained within this book. Either directly or indirectly.

Legal Notice:

This book is copyright protected. This book is only for personal use. You cannot amend, distribute, sell, use, quote or paraphrase any part, or the content within this book, without the consent of the author or publisher.

Disclaimer Notice:

Please note the information contained within this document is for educational and entertainment purpose sonly. All effort has been executed to present accurate, up to date, and reliable, complete information. No warranties of any kind are declared or implied. Readers acknowledge that the author is not engaging in the rendering of legal, financial, medical or professional advice. The content within this book has been derived from various sources. Please consult a licensed professional before attempting any techniques outlined in this book. By reading this document, the reader agrees that under no circumstances is the author responsible for any losses, direct or indirect, which are incurred as a result of the use of information contained within this document, including, but not limited to, - errors, omissions, or inaccuracies.

Copyright © 2021 Janeth Cole

All rights reserved.

ISBN: 978-1-80301-486-9 (Paperback)

ISBN: 978-1-80301-487-6 (Hardcover)

Table of Contents

Chapter 1 - Introduction 7

Chapter 2 - Breakfast Recipes 8

   1) Cheesy Red Omelette 9

   2) Apple Warm Oatmeal 9

   3) Golden Coco Mix 9

   4) Delicious Agave Rice 9

   5) Italian Feta Breakfast Eggs 9

   6) Cinnamon Pumpkin Oatmeal with Vanilla Flavour 10

   7) Button Mushroom Omelette 10

   8) Easy Tofu Bowl 10

   9) Canned Beans and Tomato Breads 10

   10) Black Olives and Feta Bread 11

   11) Lentils and Mushroom Burgers 11

   12) Cheesy Baked Potato 11

   13) Breakfast Walnuts Quinoa 11

   14) Vegetables Wraps with Soy Sauce 12

   15) Brown Rice and Chickpeas Breakfast Bowl 12

   16) Sauté Vegan Millet 12

   17) Black Navel Salad 12

   18) Almond Pearls Pudding 13

   19) Awesome Brakfast Muesli 13

   20) Delicious Kamut Salad with Walnuts .. 13

Chapter 3 - Rice & Grain and Pasta Recipes. 14

   21) Pasta with Delicious Spanish Salsa .. 15

   22) Penne with Zucchini and Wine 15

   23) Gochujang and Carrot Spaghetti with Coriander 15

   24) Spinach Cheesy Pasta 16

   25) Chickpeas Tomato Pasta with Tamari .. 16

   26) Italian Tricolor Pasta 16

   27) Fusilli with Juicy Cauliflowers 17

   28) Shrimp Fettuccine with Black Pepper . 17

   29) Spiced Kidney Pasta with Cilantro ... 17

   30) Classic Grandma's Pasta 17

   31) Red Lentils Spaghetti with Herbs 18

   32) Spicy Shrimp Pasta with Bay Scallops. 18

   33) Italian Pasta e Fagioli 18

   34) Penne with Vodka Cream 19

   35) Macaroni with Cherry and Peas 19

   36) Brown Rice with Lentils in Veggie Broth. 19

   37) Golden Rice with Pistachios 20

   38) Quinoa and Veggie Mix Salad 20

   39) Chili Bean Mix 20

   40) Bean Balls with Red pepper and Marinara Sauce 21

Chapter 4 - Side and Salad Recipes 22

   41) Veggie ChimiSalad 23

   42) Exotic Quinoa Bowl 23

   43) Linguini with Peas and Parmigiano Reggiano 23

   44) Noodles Salad with Peanut Butter Cream 24

   45) Delicious Potato Salad with Mustard . 24

   46) Easy Creamy Kernel 24

47) Green Bean with Walnut Mix 25

48) Old School Panzanella 25

49) Vegan Chorizo Salad with Red Wine Vinegar 25

50) Juicy Smoked Apple Salad 26

51) Kalamata Pepper Salad with Pine Nuts ... 26

52) Spiced Carrot Bowl 26

53) Double Green Juicy Salad 26

54) Lemony Orange Fennel Salad 27

55) Asian Goji Salad 27

56) Cheesy Asparagus Pesto Salad 27

57) Ricotta Seed Salad 27

58) Veggie Almond Chermoula Bowl 28

59) Baked Asparagus Maple Salad 28

60) Cherry Kalamata Salad with Oregano 28

Chapter 5 - Main Recipes 30

61) Zucchini Rice with Chicken Chunks 31

62) Smoked Baby Spinach Stew 31

63) Green Chilis Chicken Breast 31

64) Chicken Breast with Italian Seasoning.... 31

65) Veggie Ragù Noodles 32

66) Quinoa Chicken with Olives and Grrek Seasoning 32

67) Red Quinoa Burgers with Thaini Guacamole 32

68) Rice and Beans with Red Bell pepper 33

69) Baked Sole with Pistachos 33

70) Quinoa with Avocado and Pepper Mix 33

71) Lemony Mussels in Dry Wine Sauce 34

72) Cold Spinach with Fruit Mix 34

73) Juiced Shrimp with Herbs 34

74) Veggie Grill with Herbs and Cider Vinegar 35

75) Cheesy Gnocchi with Shrimp 35

76) Hummus Quinoa with Edamame Bowl ... 35

77) Fresh Salmon Fillet with Pepper 35

78) Delicious Puttanesca with Fresh Shrimp 36

79) Different Spicy Lasagna 36

80) Italian Green Seitan 36

Chapter 6 - Soup Recipes 38

81) Smoked Red Soup 39

82) Lettuce Egg Soup Bowl 39

83) Cayenne Kale and Mushrooms Soup 39

84) Coco Butternut Soup 39

85) Cauliflower Broth with Leek 39

86) Split Veggie Soup 40

87) Minestrone Bean Soup 40

88) Swiss Coco Whisked Egg Soup 40

89) Spinach and Mushroom Soup with Fresh Cream 40

90) Veggie Soup with Peanut Butter 41

91) Simple Red Lentil Soup 41

92) Creamy Squash Soup 41

93) Asparagus and Seed Soup with Cashew Cream 41

94) Spicy Bean Carrot and Lentil Soup 42

95) Broccoli Ginger Soup with Herbs 42

96) Creamy Kabocha Soup 42

97) Beans and Green Soup 42

98) Sweety Onion Soup 43

99) Lentils and Bean Mix in Masala Soup 43

100) Cauli Soup with Matcha Tea 43

Chapter 7 - Snack Recipe 44

101) Smoked Thaini Beets Hummus 45

102) Lemony Fava Cream 45

- 103) Zucchini Hummus with Cumin 45
- 104) Crispy Hummus Bell Pepper 45
- 105) Totopos Enchilados 45
- 106) Garlic Tomato Italian Toast 46
- 107) Spanish Potato Tortillas 46
- 108) Turkish Delicious Spiced Falafel 46
- 109) Red Pesto Bruschetta 46
- 110) Cheesy Low-Fat Yogurt Dip 47
- 111) Exotic Hummus And Sprout Toast 47
- 112) Rich Ricotta Snack 47
- 113) Sweety Apple Toast with Cinnamon ... 47
- 114) Crispy Zucchini 47
- 115) Summer Vegetarian Wraps 48
- 116) Spiced Pineapple Mix 48
- 117) Salmon Wraps with Balsamic Vinegar 48
- 118) Incredible Dried Snack 48
- 119) Crispy Beet with Rosemary 49
- 120) Sweety Oats with Cinnamon 49

Chapter 8 - Dessert and Smoothie Recipes ... 50

- 121) Cocoflakes Cantaloupe Yogurt with Raspberry 51
- 122) Plant-Based Berry and Banana Smoothie 51
- 123) Delicious Apple Compote with Cinnamon 51
- 124) Carrot and Prunes Smoothie with Walnuts 51
- 125) Choco Bombs 51
- 126) Dark Date and Banana Drink 51
- 127) Sweety Watermelon Iced Flakes 52
- 128) Cashew and Fruit Mix Smoothie 52
- 129) Seed Butter Cookies 52
- 130) Persimmon Healthy Smoothie 52
- 131) Sweety Rice with Rose Water and Dried Figs 52
- 132) Fresh and Dry Smoothie 53
- 133) Greek Yogurt with Honey and Fruit Mix 53
- 134) Almond Berries and Banana Smoothie 53
- 135) Choco Walnuts Cube with Thaini 53
- 136) Fruit Explosion Smoothie 53
- 137) Greek Granola Berries 53
- 138) Energy Almond Smoothie 54
- 139) Figs and Walnuts with Honey Topping 54
- 140) Thaini Figs Smoothie 54

Chapter 9 - Simple Dr. Cole's Meal Plan – For Women 55

Chapter 10 - Conclusion 57

Chapter 1 - Introduction

The Dietary Approaches to Stop Hypertension better known as the DASH diet is more than a fad or a trend, it can really make a difference in your health and your appearance. In contrast to other diets, the DASH diet emerged from a group of specialists in 1997 with the goal of reducing high blood pressure. Later, other benefits were found, including the prevention of type II diabetes and help during menopause.

In a research conducted by Valentino, Giovanna, Tagle, Rodrigo, & Acevedo, Mónica (2014) mention the benefits of DASH diet during menopause as a treatment that mitigates the effects caused by the decrease in estrogen production.

Dash Diet Manifesto

The central manifesto of the DASH diet is to reduce dietary sodium to below 2.3 g in regular DASH and 1.5 g in low sodium DASH (equivalent to 3.8 g of salt); increasing consumption of foods rich in potassium, calcium, fiber and magnesium.

In simple terms, it consists of reducing the intake of salt, fats and sugars as much as possible.

What foods can I eat on the DASH diet?

The first thing you should consider is the reduction or elimination of fatty foods, sugary or processed products. You should increase your intake of fresh fruits and vegetables, nuts and seeds, whole grains and dried fruits, fish and lean meat, low-fat or fat-free dairy products. For cooking or frying your food you can opt for olive, coconut or soybean oil.

It also encourages you to stay hydrated by drinking 2 liters of water daily, which also allows you to eliminate excess sodium. Use low-fat cooking techniques such as grilling, broiling, roasting, baking, microwaving or steaming cooking.

Benefits to women

There are many benefits of the DASH diet for all women no matter what age or stage of life you are in, for example: it is your ally during menopause and pre-menopause, helps you lose weight, controls high blood pressure, prevents type II diabetes, reduces the risk of heart disease, controls and improves cholesterol levels, prevents the development of annoying kidney stones. Discover that eating smart is the best way to a fit and healthy body.

Valentino, Giovanna, Tagle, Rodrigo, & Acevedo, Mónica. (2014). Dieta DASH y menopausia: Más allá de los beneficios en hipertensión arterial. *Revista chilena de cardiología, 33*(3), 215-222. https://dx.doi.org/10.4067/S0718-85602014000300008

Chapter 2 -   Breakfast Recipes

1) Cheesy Red Omelette

Preparation Time: 5 minutes

Cooking Time: 10 minutes

Servings: 4

Nutrition: Calories: 191 Fat: 15g Carbs: 6g Protein: 9g

Ingredients:
- 2 tablespoons olive oil
- 1 medium onion, chopped
- 1 teaspoon garlic, minced
- 2 medium tomatoes, chopped
- 6 large eggs
- ½ cup half and half
- ½ cup feta cheese, crumbled
- ¼ cup dill weed
- Ground black pepper as needed

Directions:
- Pre-heat your oven to a temperature of 400 degrees Fahrenheit. Take a large sized ovenproof pan and heat up your olive oil over medium-high heat. Toss in the onion, garlic, tomatoes and stir fry them for 4 minutes.
- While they are being cooked, take a bowl and beat together your eggs, half and half cream and season the mix with some pepper.
- Pour the mixture into the pan with your vegetables and top it with crumbled feta cheese and dill weed. Cover it with the lid and let it cook for 3 minutes.
- Place the pan inside your oven and let it bake for 10 minutes. Serve hot.

2) Apple Warm Oatmeal

Preparation Time: 10 minutes

Cooking Time: 4 minutes

Servings: 3

Nutrition: calories 200, fat 1g, carbs 12g, protein 10g

Ingredients:
- 3 cups water
- 1 cup steel cut oats
- 1 apple, cored and chopped
- 1 tablespoon cinnamon powder

Directions:
- In your instant pot, mix water with oats, cinnamon and apple, stir, cover and Cooking Time: on High for 4 minutes.
- Stir again, divide into bowls and serve for breakfast.
- Enjoy!

3) Golden Coco Mix

Preparation Time: 15 minutes

Cooking Time: 0 minutes

Servings: 6

Nutrition: Calories: 259 Fat: 13g Carbs: 5g Protein: 16g

Ingredients:
- Powdered erythritol as needed
- 1 ½ cups almond milk, unsweetened
- 2 tablespoons vanilla protein powder
- 3 tablespoons Golden Flaxseed meal
- 2 tablespoons coconut flour

Directions:
- Take a bowl and mix in flaxseed meal, protein powder, coconut flour and mix well. Add mix to saucepan (placed over medium heat).
- Add almond milk and stir, let the mixture thicken. Add your desired amount of sweetener and serve. Enjoy!

4) Delicious Agave Rice

Preparation Time: 10 minutes

Cooking Time: 7 minutes

Servings: 4

Nutrition: calories 192, fat 1g, carbs 20g, protein 4g

Ingredients:
- 1 cup Arborio rice
- 2 cups almond milk
- 1 cup coconut milk
- 1/3 cup agave nectar
- 2 teaspoons vanilla extract
- ¼ cup coconut flakes, toasted

Directions:
- Set your instant pot on simmer mode, add almond and coconut milk and bring to a boil.
- Add agave nectar and rice, stir, cover and Cooking Time: on High for 5 minutes.
- Add vanilla and coconut, stir, divide into bowls and serve warm.
- Enjoy!

5) Italian Feta Breakfast Eggs

Preparation Time: 5 minutes

Cooking Time: 15 minutes

Servings: 12

Nutrition: Calories: 106 Fat: 8g Carbs: 2g Protein: 7g

Ingredients:
- 2 tablespoons of unsalted butter (replace with canola oil for full effect)
- ½ cup of chopped up scallions
- 1 cup of crumbled feta cheese
- 8 large sized eggs
- 2/3 cup of milk
- ½ teaspoon of dried Italian seasoning
- Freshly ground black pepper as needed
- Cooking oil spray

Directions:
- Pre-heat your oven to 400 degrees Fahrenheit. Take a 3-4 ounce muffin pan and grease with cooking oil. Take a non-stick pan and place it over medium heat.
- Add butter and allow the butter to melt. Add half of the scallions and stir fry. Keep them to the side. Take a medium-sized bowl and add eggs, Italian seasoning and milk and whisk well.
- Add the stir fried scallions and feta cheese and mix. Season with pepper. Pour the mix into the muffin tin. Transfer the muffin tin to your oven and bake for 15 minutes. Serve with a sprinkle of scallions.

6) Cinnamon Pumpkin Oatmeal with Vanilla Flavour

Preparation Time: 10 minutes

Cooking Time: 3 minutes

Servings: 6

Nutrition: calories 173, fat 1g, carbs 20g, protein 6g

Ingredients:
- 4 and ½ cups water
- 1 and ½ cups steel cut oats
- 2 teaspoons cinnamon powder
- 1 teaspoon vanilla extract
- 1 teaspoon allspice
- 1 and ½ cup pumpkin puree
- ¼ cup pecans, chopped

Directions:
- In your instant pot, mix water with oats, cinnamon, vanilla allspice and pumpkin puree, stir, cover and Cooking Time: on High for 3 minutes.
- Divide into bowls, stir again, cool down and serve with pecans on top.
- Enjoy!

7) Button Mushroom Omelette

Preparation Time: 5 minutes

Cooking Time: 15 minutes

Servings: 4

Nutrition: Calories: 189 **Fat:** 13g **Carbs:** 6g **Protein:** 12g

Ingredients:
- 2 tablespoons of butter (replace with canola oil for full effect)
- 1 chopped up medium-sized onion
- 2 minced cloves of garlic
- 1 cup of coarsely chopped baby rocket tomato
- 1 cup of sliced button mushrooms
- 6 large pieces of eggs
- ½ cup of skim milk
- 1 teaspoon of dried rosemary
- Ground black pepper as needed

Directions:
- Pre-heat your oven to 400 degrees Fahrenheit. Take a large oven-proof pan and place it over medium-heat. Heat up some oil.
- Stir fry your garlic, onion for about 2 minutes. Add the mushroom, rosemary and rockets and cook for 3 minutes. Take a medium-sized bowl and beat your eggs alongside the milk.
- Season it with some pepper. Pour the egg mixture into your pan with the vegetables and sprinkle some Parmesan.
- Reduce the heat to low and cover with the lid. Let it cook for 3 minutes. Transfer the pan into your oven and bake for 10 minutes until fully settled.
- Reduce the heat to low and cover with your lid. Let it cook for 3 minutes. Transfer the pan into your oven and then bake for another 10 minutes. Serve hot.

8) Easy Tofu Bowl

Preparation Time: 10 minutes

Cooking Time: 10 minutes

Servings: 4

Nutrition: calories 172, fat 7g, carbs 20g, protein 6g

Ingredients:
- 1 pound extra firm tofu, cubed
- 1 cup sweet potato, chopped
- 3 garlic cloves, minced
- 2 tablespoons sesame seeds
- 1 yellow onion, chopped
- 2 teaspoons sesame seed oil
- 1 carrot, chopped
- 1 tablespoon tamari
- 1 tablespoon rice vinegar
- 2 cups snow peas, halved
- 1/3 cup veggie stock
- 2 tablespoons red pepper sauce
- 2 tablespoons scallions, chopped
- 2 tablespoons tahini paste

Directions:
- Set your instant pot on sauté mode, add oil, heat it up, add sweet potato, onion and carrots, stir and Cooking Time: for 2 minutes.
- Add garlic, half of the sesame seeds, tofu, vinegar, tamari and stock, stir and Cooking Time: for 2 minutes more.
- Cover pot and Cooking Time: on High for 3 minutes more.
- Add peas, the rest of the sesame seeds, green onions, tahini paste and pepper sauce, stir, cover and Cooking Time: on Low for 1 minutes more.
- Divide into bowls and serve for breakfast.
- Enjoy!

9) Canned Beans and Tomato Breads

Preparation Time: 5 minutes

Cooking Time: 15 minutes

Servings: 4

Nutrition: Calories 382 **Fat:** 1.8g **Carbs:** 66g **Protein:** 28.5g

Ingredients:
- 1 ½ tbsp olive oil
- 1 tomato, cubed
- 1 garlic clove, minced
- 1 red onion, chopped
- ¼ cup parsley, chopped
- 15 oz. canned fava beans, drained and rinsed
- ¼ cup lemon juice
- Black pepper to the taste
- 4 whole-wheat pita bread pockets

Directions:
- Heat a pan with the oil over medium heat, add the onion, stir, and sauté for 5 minutes. Add the rest of the ingredients, stir, and cook for 10 minutes more
- Stuff the pita pockets with this mix and serve for breakfast.

10) Black Olives and Feta Bread

Preparation Time: 1 hour and 40 minutes

Cooking Time: 30 minutes

Servings: 10

Nutrition: Calories 251 Fat: 7.3g Carbs: 39.7g Protein: 6.7g

Ingredients:
- 4 cups whole-wheat flour
- 3 tbsps. oregano, chopped
- 2 tsps. dry yeast
- ¼ cup olive oil
- 1 ½ cups black olives, pitted and sliced
- 1 cup of water
- ½ cup feta cheese, crumbled

Directions:
- In a bowl, mix the flour with the water, the yeast, and the oil. Stir and knead your dough very well. Put the dough in a bowl, cover with plastic wrap, and keep in a warm place for 1 hour.
- Divide the dough into 2 bowls and stretch each ball well. Add the rest of the ingredients to each ball and tuck them inside. Knead the dough well again.
- Flatten the balls a bit and leave them aside for 40 minutes more. Transfer the balls to a baking sheet lined with parchment paper, make a small slit in each, and bake at 425F for 30 minutes.
- Serve the bread as a Mediterranean breakfast.

11) Lentils and Mushroom Burgers

Preparation Time: 10 minutes

Cooking Time: 30 minutes

Servings: 4

Nutrition: calories 140, fat 3g, carbs 14g, protein 13g

Ingredients:
- 1 cup mushrooms, chopped
- 2 teaspoons ginger, grated
- 1 cup yellow onion, chopped
- 1 cup red lentils
- 1 sweet potato, chopped
- 2 and ½ cups veggie stock
- ¼ cup hemp seeds
- ¼ cup parsley, chopped
- 1 tablespoon curry powder
- ¼ cup cilantro, chopped
- 1 cup quick oats
- 4 tablespoons rice flour

Direction:
- Set your instant pot on sauté mode, add onion, mushrooms and ginger, stir and sauté for 2 minutes.
- Add lentils, stock and sweet potatoes, stir, cover and Cooking Time: on High for 6 minutes.
- Leave this mixture aside to cool down, mash using a potato masher, add parsley, hemp, curry powder, cilantro, oats and rice flour and stir well.
- Shape 8 patties out of this mix, arrange them all on a lined baking sheet, introduce in the oven at 375 degrees F and bake for 10 minutes on each side.
- Divide between plates and serve for breakfast.
- Enjoy!

12) Cheesy Baked Potato

Preparation Time: 10 minutes

Cooking Time: 1 hour and 10 minutes

Servings: 8

Nutrition: Calories 476 Fat: 16.8g Carbs: 68.8g Protein: 13.9g

Ingredients:
- 2 pounds sweet potatoes, peeled and cubed
- ¼ cup olive oil + a drizzle
- 7 oz. feta cheese, crumbled
- 1 yellow onion, chopped
- 2 eggs, whisked
- ¼ cup almond milk
- 1 tbsp. herbs de Provence
- A pinch of black pepper
- 6 phyllo sheets
- 1 tbsp. parmesan, grated

Directions:
- In a bowl, combine the potatoes with half of the oil, and pepper, toss, spread on a baking sheet lined with parchment paper, and roast at 400F for 25 minutes.
- Meanwhile, heat a pan with half of the remaining oil over medium heat, add the onion, and sauté for 5 minutes.
- In a bowl, combine the eggs with the milk, feta, herbs, pepper, onion, sweet potatoes, and the rest of the oil and toss.
- Arrange the phyllo sheets in a tart pan and brush them with a drizzle of oil. Add the sweet potato mix and spread it well into the pan.
- Sprinkle the parmesan on top and bake covered with tin foil at 350F for 20 minutes. Remove the tin foil, bake the tart for 20 minutes more, cool it down, slice, and serve for breakfast.

13) Breakfast Walnuts Quinoa

Preparation Time: 5 minutes

Cooking Time: 0 minutes

Servings: 4

Nutrition: Calories 284 Fat: 14.3g Carbs: 15.4g Protein: 4.4g

Ingredients:
- 2 cups almond milk
- 2 cups quinoa, already cooked
- ½ tsp cinnamon powder
- 1 tbsp. honey
- 1 cup blueberries
- ¼ cup walnuts, chopped

Directions:
- In a bowl, mix the quinoa with the milk and the rest of the ingredients, toss, divide into smaller bowls and serve for breakfast

14) Vegetables Wraps with Soy Sauce

Preparation Time: 10 minutes

Cooking Time: 15 minutes

Servings: 6

Nutrition: calories 100, fat 2g, carbs 9g, protein 3g

Ingredients:
- 1 tablespoon olive oil
- 1 cup mushrooms, chopped
- 1 and ½ cups cabbage, chopped
- ½ cup carrots, grated
- 1 and ½ cups water
- 2 tablespoons soy sauce
- 1 teaspoon ginger, grated
- 1 tablespoon rice wine vinegar
- 1 teaspoon sesame oil
- 12 vegan dumpling wrappers

Directions:
- Set your instant pot on sauté mode, add olive oil, heat it up, add mushrooms, stir and Cooking Time: for 2 minutes.
- Add carrot, cabbage, soy sauce and vinegar, stir and Cooking Time: for 3 minutes more.
- Add sesame oil and ginger, stir and transfer everything to a bowl.
- Arrange all wrappers on a working surface, divide veggie mix, wrap them and seal with some water.
- Add the water to your instant pot, add steamer basket, add dumplings inside, cover pot and Cooking Time: on High for 7 minutes.
- Divide between plates and serve for breakfast.
- Enjoy!

15) Brown Rice and Chickpeas Breakfast Bowl

Preparation Time: Breakfast Rice Bowl

Cooking Time: 30 minutes

Servings: 4

Nutrition: calories 292, fat 4g, carbs 9g, protein 10g

Ingredients:
- 1 tablespoon olive oil
- 2 tablespoons chana masala
- 1 red onion, chopped
- 1 tablespoon ginger, grated
- 1 tablespoon garlic, minced
- 1 cup chickpeas
- 3 cups water
- A pinch of black pepper
- 14 ounces tomatoes, chopped
- 1 and ½ cups brown rice

Directions:
- Set your instant pot on sauté mode, add the oil, heat it up, add onion, stir and Cooking Time: for 7 minutes.
- Add pepper, chana masala, ginger and garlic, stir and Cooking Time: for 1
- minute more.
- Add tomatoes, chickpeas, rice and water, stir, cover and Cooking Time: on High for 20 minutes.
- Stir one more time, divide into bowls and serve for breakfast.
- Enjoy!

16) Sauté Vegan Millet

Preparation Time: 10 minutes

Cooking Time: 16 minutes

Servings: 4

Nutrition: calories 172, fat 3g, carbs 19g, protein 5g

Ingredients:
- 1 cup millet
- ½ cup oyster mushrooms, chopped
- 2 garlic cloves, minced
- ½ cup green lentils
- ½ cup bok choy, chopped
- 2 and ¼ cups veggie stock
- 1 cup yellow onion, chopped
- 1 cup asparagus, chopped
- 1 tablespoon lemon juice
- ¼ cup parsley and chives, chopped

Directions:
- Set your instant pot on sauté mode, heat it up, add garlic, onion and mushrooms, stir and Cooking Time: for 2 minutes.
- Add lentils and millet, stir and Cooking Time: for a few seconds more.
- Add stock, stir, cover and Cooking Time: on High for 10 minutes.
- Add asparagus and bok choy, stir, cover and leave everything aside for 3 minutes.
- Add parsley and chives and lemon juice, stir, divide into bowls and serve for breakfast.
- Enjoy!

17) Black Navel Salad

Preparation Time: 5 minutes

Cooking Time: 0 minutes

Servings: 4

Nutrition: Calories 97 Fat: 9.1g Carbs: 3.7g Protein: 1.9g

Ingredients:
- 1 tbsp. balsamic vinegar
- 2 garlic cloves, minced
- 1 tsp. Dijon mustard
- 2 tbsps. olive oil
- 1 tbsp. lemon juice
- Black pepper to taste
- ½ cup black olives, pitted and chopped
- 1 tbsp. parsley, chopped
- 7 cups baby spinach
- 2 endives, shredded
- 3 medium navel oranges, peeled and cut into segments
- 2 bulbs fennel, shredded

Directions:
- In a salad bowl, combine the spinach with the endives, oranges, fennel, and the rest of the ingredients, toss and serve for breakfast.

18) Almond Pearls Pudding

Preparation Time: 10 minutes

Cooking Time: 8 minutes

Servings: 4

Nutrition: calories 187, fat 3g, fiber 1g, carbs 18g, protein 3g

Ingredients:
- 1/3 cup tapioca pearls
- ½ cup water
- 1 and ¼ cups almond milk
- ½ cup stevia
- Zest from ½ lemon, grated

Directions:
- In a heatproof bowl, mix tapioca with almond milk, stevia and lemon zest and stir well.
- Add the water to your instant pot, add steamer basket, and heatproof bowl inside, cover and Cooking Time: on High for 8 minutes.
- Stir your pudding and serve for breakfast.
- Enjoy!

19) Awesome Brakfast Muesli

Preparation Time: 15 minutes

Cooking Time: 20 minutes

Servings: 8

Nutrition: Calories 250 Fat: 10g Carbs: 36g Protein: 7g

Ingredients:
- 3 ½ cups rolled oats
- ½ cup wheat bran
- ½ tsp ground cinnamon
- ½ cup sliced almonds
- ¼ cup raw pecans, coarsely chopped
- ¼ cup raw pepitas (shelled pumpkin seeds)
- ½ cup unsweetened coconut flakes
- ¼ cup dried apricots, coarsely chopped
- ¼ cup dried cherries

Directions:
- Take a medium bowl and combine the oats, wheat bran and cinnamon. Stir well. Place the mixture onto a baking sheet.
- Next place the almonds, pecans, and pepitas onto another baking sheet and toss. Pop both trays into the oven and heat to 350°F. Bake for 10-12 minutes. Remove from the oven and pop to one side.
- Leave the nuts to cool but take the one with the oats, sprinkle with the coconut, and pop back into the oven for 5 minutes more. Remove and leave to cool.
- Find a large bowl and combine the contents of both trays then stir well to combine. Throw in the apricots and cherries and stir well. Pop into an airtight container until required.

20) Delicious Kamut Salad with Walnuts

Preparation Time: 10 minutes

Cooking Time: 15 minutes

Servings: 6

Nutrition: calories 125, fat 6g, fiber 2g, carbs 4g, protein 3g

Ingredients:
- 2 cups water
- 1 cup kamut grains, soaked for 12 hours, drained and mixed with some lemon juice
- 1 teaspoon sunflower oil
- 4 ounces arugula
- 2 blood oranges, peeled and cut into medium segments
- 1 tablespoon olive oil
- 3 ounces walnuts, chopped

Directions:
- In your instant pot, mix kamut grains with sunflower oil and the water, stir, cover and Cooking Time: on High for 15 minutes.
- Drain kamut, transfer to a bowl, add a
- pinch of salt, arugula, orange segments, oil and walnuts, toss well and serve for breakfast.
- Enjoy!

Chapter 3 -   Rice & Grain and Pasta Recipes

21) *Pasta with Delicious Spanish Salsa*

Preparation Time: 15 minutes

Cooking Time:

Servings: 2

Nutrition: Carbs: 69g Protein: 12.7g Fats: 2.3g Calories: 364

Ingredients:
- Spaghetti : 160g
- Red onion: ½ roughly chopped
- Green pepper: 1 chopped
- Cherry tomatoes:250g
- Tabasco: a good dash
- Garlic: ½ clove
- Vinegar: 1 tbsp
- Basi l a small bunch

Directions:
- Cooking Time: pasta as per packet instructions
- In the meanwhile, take a blender and add tomatoes, garlic, onion, and pepper, and blend
- Add in Tabasco and vinegar and combine well
- Add the sauce to the paste
- Top with basil and serve

22) *Penne with Zucchini and Wine*

Preparation Time: 15 minutes

Cooking Time: 30 minutes

Servings: 6

Nutrition: Calories: 340 Fat: 6.2g Protein: 8.0g Carbs: 66.8g

Ingredients:
- 1 large zucchini, diced
- 1 large butternut squash, peeled and diced
- 1 large yellow onion, chopped
- 2 tablespoons extra-virgin olive oil
- 1 teaspoon paprika
- ½ teaspoon garlic powder
- ½ teaspoon freshly ground black pepper
- 1 pound (454 g) whole-grain penne
- ½ cup dry white wine
- 2 tablespoons grated Parmesan cheese

Directions:
- Preheat the oven to 400°F (205°C). Line a baking sheet with aluminum foil. Combine the zucchini, butternut squash, and onion in a large bowl.
- Drizzle with olive oil and sprinkle with paprika, garlic powder, and ground black pepper. Toss to coat well.
- Spread the vegetables in the single layer on the baking sheet, then roast in the preheated oven for 25 minutes or until the vegetables are tender.
- Meanwhile, bring a pot of water to a boil, then add the penne and cook for 14 minutes or until al dente. Drain the penne through a colander.
- Transfer ½ cup of roasted vegetables in a food processor, then pour in the dry white wine. Pulse until smooth.
- Pour the puréed vegetables in a nonstick skillet and cook with penne over medium-high heat for a few minutes to heat through.
- Transfer the penne with the purée on a large serving plate, then spread the remaining roasted vegetables and Parmesan on top before serving.

23) *Gochujang and Carrot Spaghetti with Coriander*

Preparation Time: 45 minutes

Cooking Time:

Servings: 2

Nutrition: Carbs: 52.5g Protein: 10.9g Fats: 15.5g Calories: 404

Ingredients:
- Spaghetti: 2 cups
- Olive oil: 2 tbsp
- Cauliflower: 2 cups cut in big florets
- Gochujang: 2 tbsp
- Rice vinegar: 1 tbsp
- Sliced red pepper: 1 cup sliced
- Carrot: 2 sliced
- Pepper: as per your taste
- Coriander: 1/2 cup chopped

Directions:
- Cooking Time: spaghetti as per packet instructions
- Preheat the oven 200C
- Add cauliflowers to the baking sheet and sprinkle seasoning and brush with olive oil
- Roast for 25 minutes till it turns golden and soft
- Remove from oven and brush with gochujang and Cooking Time: in the oven again for 10 minutes
- Add to the bowl and mix with carrots and red bell pepper
- Season with coriander, and pepper and pour vinegar from top
- Spread spaghetti on the serving tray and top with the cauliflower

24) Spinach Cheesy Pasta

Preparation Time: 15 minutes

Cooking Time: 14-16 minutes

Servings: 4

Nutrition: Calories: 262 Fat: 4.0g Protein: 15.0g Carbs: 51.0g

Ingredients:
- 8 ounces (227 g) uncooked penne
- 1 tablespoon extra-virgin olive oil
- 2 garlic cloves, minced
- ¼ teaspoon crushed red pepper
- 2 cups chopped fresh flat-leaf parsley, including stems
- 5 cups loosely packed baby spinach
- ¼ teaspoon ground nutmeg
- ¼ teaspoon freshly ground black pepper
- 1/3 cup Castelvetrano olives, pitted and sliced
- 1/3 cup grated Parmesan cheese

Directions:
- In a large stockpot of salted water, cook the pasta for about 8 to 10 minutes. Drain the pasta and reserve ¼ cup of the cooking liquid.
- Meanwhile, heat the olive oil in a large skillet over medium heat. Add the garlic and red pepper and cook for 30 seconds, stirring constantly.
- Add the parsley and cook for 1 minute, stirring constantly. Add the spinach, nutmeg and pepper, and cook for 3 minutes, stirring occasionally, or until the spinach is wilted.
- Add the cooked pasta and the reserved ¼ cup cooking liquid to the skillet. Stir in the olives and cook for about 2 minutes, or until most of the pasta water has been absorbed.
- Remove from the heat and stir in the cheese before serving.

25) Chickpeas Tomato Pasta with Tamari

Preparation Time: 30 minutes

Cooking Time:

Servings: 2

Nutrition: Carbs: 54g Protein: 14.6g Fats: 18g Calories: 442

Ingredients:
- Pasta: 1 cup cooked
- Chickpeas: 1 cup rinsed and drained well
- Onion: 1 cup finely diced
- Tomato: 2 cups diced
- Lemon juice: 2 tbsp
- Kale: 1 cup
- Olive oil: 2 tbsp
- Tamari: 1 tbsp
- Coriander: 2 tbsp chopped
- Garlic: 1 clove crushed

Directions:
- Cooking Time: pasta as per packet instructions
- Add garlic, lemon juice, tamari, and olive oil in a bowl and whisk
- Take a serving bowl and combine kale, pasta, chickpeas, onion, tomatoes, and the sauce you made
- Add coriander from the top and serve

26) Italian Tricolor Pasta

Preparation Time: 5 minutes

Cooking Time: 25 minutes

Servings: 6

Nutrition: Calories: 147 Fat: 3.0g Protein: 16.0g Carbs: 17.0g

Ingredients:
- 8 ounces (227 g) uncooked small pasta, like orecchiette (little ears) or farfalle (bow ties)
- 1½ pounds (680 g) fresh asparagus, ends trimmed and stalks chopped into 1-inch pieces
- 1½ cups grape tomatoes, halved
- 2 tablespoons extra-virgin olive oil
- ¼ teaspoon freshly ground black pepper
- 2 cups fresh Mozzarella, drained and cut into bite-size pieces (about 8 ounces / 227 g)
- 1/3 cup torn fresh basil leaves
- 2 tablespoons balsamic vinegar

Directions:
- Preheat the oven to 400°F (205°C). In a large stockpot of salted water, cook the pasta for about 8 to 10 minutes. Drain and reserve about ¼ cup of the cooking liquid.
- Meanwhile, in a large bowl, toss together the asparagus, tomatoes, oil and pepper. Spread the mixture onto a large, rimmed baking sheet and bake in the oven for 15 minutes, stirring twice during cooking.
- Remove the vegetables from the oven and add the cooked pasta to the baking sheet. Mix with a few tablespoons of cooking liquid to help the sauce become smoother and the saucy vegetables stick to the pasta.
- Gently mix in the Mozzarella and basil. Drizzle with the balsamic vinegar. Serve from the baking sheet or pour the pasta into a large bowl.

27) Fusilli with Juicy Cauliflowers

Preparation Time: 20 minutes

Cooking Time:

Servings: 2

Nutrition: Carbs: 21.6g Protein: 4.85g Fats: 7.9g Calories: 172

Ingredients:
- Fusilli: 1 cup cooked
- Cauliflower: 1 cup roughly chopped
- Garlic: 2 cloves thinly sliced
- Olive oil: 1 tbsp
- Chili flakes: 1 tsp
- Pepper: as per your taste
- Lemon: 1 juice and zest

Directions:
- Cooking Time: the pasta as per the packet instruction
- Add cauliflower when the pasta is about to be done
- Drain but keep one cup of the water
- Take a large pan and heat oil
- Add in garlic and Cooking Time: for two minutes
- Add in chili and Cooking Time: for a minutes
- Add pasta, lemon juice and zest, pepper, and cauliflower with the pasta water
- Mix everything well and serve

28) Shrimp Fettuccine with Black Pepper

Preparation Time: 15 minutes

Cooking Time: 15 minutes

Servings: 4-6

Nutrition: Calories: 615 Fat: 17.0g Protein: 33.0g Carbs: 89.0g

Ingredients:
- 8 ounces (227 g) fettuccine pasta
- ¼ cup extra-virgin olive oil
- 3 tablespoons garlic, minced
- 1 pound (454 g) large shrimp, peeled and deveined
- 1/3 cup lemon juice
- 1 tablespoon lemon zest
- ½ teaspoon freshly ground black pepper

Directions:
- Bring a large pot of water to a boil. Add the fettuccine and cook for 8 minutes. Reserve ½ cup of the cooking liquid and drain the pasta.
- In a large saucepan over medium heat, heat the olive oil. Add the garlic and sauté for 1 minute.
- Add the shrimp to the saucepan and cook each side for 3 minutes. Remove the shrimp from the pan and set aside.
- Add the remaining ingredients to the saucepan. Stir in the cooking liquid. Add the pasta and toss together to evenly coat the pasta.
- Transfer the pasta to a serving dish and serve topped with the cooked shrimp.

29) Spiced Kidney Pasta with Cilantro

Preparation Time: 30 minutes

Cooking Time:

Servings: 4

Nutrition: Carbs: 41.98g Protein: 9.3g Fats: 8.4g Calories: 274

Ingredients:
- Pasta: 2 cups (after cooking
- Onion: 1 chopped
- Garlic: 1 ½ tsp minced
- Cumin: 1 tsp
- Frozen corn: 1 cup
- Cayenne pepper: ¼ tsp
- Kidney beans: 1 cup drained and rinsed
- Fresh cilantro: 2 tsp
- Lemon juice: 3 tbsp
- Cooking oil: 2 tbsp

Directions:
- Cooking Time: pasta as per packet instructions
- Take a saucepan and heat oil in it
- Add garlic and onion to it and make them tender
- Add cayenne pepper, and cumin
- Now add corns and beans and mix well
- Cover and Cooking Time: for 5 minutes
- Add in pasta and stir and remove from heat after 5 minutes
- Pour lemon juice on top
- Garnish with cilantro and serve

30) Classic Grandma's Pasta

Preparation Time: 15 minutes

Cooking Time: 25 minutes

Servings: 4

Nutrition: Calories 500 Fat 18.3 g Carbohydrates 69.7 g Protein 16.2 g

Ingredients:
- 1 pack of 16 angel hair pasta
- 1/4 cup of olive oil
- 1/2 onion, minced
- 4 cloves of chopped garlic
- 2 cups of Roma tomatoes, diced
- 2 tablespoons balsamic vinegar
- 1 low-sodium chicken broth
- ground red pepper
- freshly ground black pepper to taste
- 1/4 cup grated Parmesan cheese
- 2 tablespoons chopped fresh basil

Directions:
- Bring a large pot of water to a boil. Add pasta and cook for 8 minutes or until al dente; drain.
- Pour the olive oil in a large deep pan over high heat. Fry onions and garlic until light brown. Lower the heat to medium and add tomatoes, vinegar, and chicken stock; simmer for about 8 minutes.
- Stir in the red pepper, black pepper, basil, and cooked pasta and mix well with the sauce. Simmer for about 5 minutes and serve garnished with grated cheese.

37) Golden Rice with Pistachios

Preparation Time: 5 minutes

Cooking Time: 15 minutes

Servings: 6

Nutrition: Calories: 320 Fat: 7g Carbs: 61g Protein: 6g

Ingredients:
- 1 tablespoon extra-virgin olive oil
- 1 cup chopped onion (about ½ medium onion)
- ½ cup shredded carrot (about 1 medium carrot)
- 1 teaspoon ground cumin
- ½ teaspoon ground cinnamon
- 2 cups instant brown rice
- 1¾ cups 100% orange juice
- ¼ cup water
- 1 cup golden raisins
- ½ cup shelled pistachios
- Chopped fresh chives (optional)

Directions:
- In a medium saucepan over medium-high heat, heat the oil. Add the onion and cook for 5 minutes, stirring frequently.
- Add the carrot, cumin, and cinnamon, and cook for 1 minute, stirring frequently. Stir in the rice, orange juice, and water.
- Bring to a boil, cover, then lower the heat to medium-low. Simmer for 7 minutes, or until the rice is cooked through and the liquid is absorbed. Stir in the raisins, pistachios, and chives (if using) and serve.

38) Quinoa and Veggie Mix Salad

Preparation Time: 15 minutes

Cooking Time: 15 minutes

Servings: 4

Nutrition: Calories: 366 Fat: 11.1g Protein: 15.5g Carbs: 55.6g

Ingredients:
- 1 cup red dry quinoa, rinsed and drained
- 2 cups low-sodium vegetable soup
- 2 cups fresh spinach
- 2 cups finely shredded red cabbage
- 1 (15-ounce / 425-g) can chickpeas, drained and rinsed
- 1 ripe avocado, thinly sliced
- 1 cup shredded carrots
- 1 red bell pepper, thinly sliced
- 4 tablespoons Mango Sauce
- ½ cup fresh cilantro, chopped
- Mango Sauce:
- 1 mango, diced
- ¼ cup fresh lime juice
- ½ teaspoon ground turmeric
- 1 teaspoon finely minced fresh ginger
- Pinch of ground red pepper
- 1 teaspoon pure maple syrup
- 2 tablespoons extra-virgin olive oil

Directions:
- Pour the quinoa and vegetable soup in a saucepan. Bring to a boil. Reduce the heat to low. Cover and cook for 15 minutes or until tender. Fluffy with a fork.
- Meanwhile, combine the ingredients for the mango sauce in a food processor. Pulse until smooth.
- Divide the quinoa, spinach, and cabbage into 4 serving bowls, then top with chickpeas, avocado, carrots, and bell pepper.
- Dress them with the mango sauce and spread with cilantro. Serve immediately.

39) Chili Bean Mix

Preparation Time: 15 minutes

Cooking Time: 5 hours

Servings: 4

Nutrition: Calories: 633 Fat: 16.3g Protein: 31.7g Carbs: 97.0g

Ingredients:
- 1 (28-ounce / 794-g) can chopped tomatoes, with the juice
- 1 (15-ounce / 425-g) can black beans, drained and rinsed
- 1 (15-ounce / 425-g) can redly beans, drained and rinsed
- 1 medium green bell pepper, chopped
- 1 yellow onion, chopped
- 1 tablespoon onion powder
- 1 teaspoon paprika
- 1 teaspoon cayenne pepper
- 1 teaspoon garlic powder
- ½ teaspoon ground black pepper
- 1 tablespoon olive oil
- 1 large hass avocado, pitted, peeled, and chopped, for garnish

Directions:
- Combine all the ingredients, except for the avocado, in the slow cooker. Stir to mix well.
- Put the slow cooker lid on and cook on high for 5 hours or until the vegetables are tender and the mixture has a thick consistency.
- Pour the chili in a large serving bowl. Allow to cool for 30 minutes, then spread with chopped avocado and serve.

40) Bean Balls with Red pepper and Marinara Sauce

Preparation Time: 15 minutes

Cooking Time: 30 minutes

Servings: 2-4

Nutrition: Calories: 351 Fat: 16.4g Protein: 11.5g Carbs: 42.9g

Ingredients:

Bean Balls:
- 1 tablespoon extra-virgin olive oil
- ½ yellow onion, minced
- 1 teaspoon fennel seeds
- 2 teaspoons dried oregano
- ½ teaspoon crushed red pepper flakes
- 1 teaspoon garlic powder
- 1 (15-ounce / 425-g) can white beans (cannellini or navy), drained and rinsed
- ½ cup whole-grain bread crumbs
- Ground black pepper, to taste

Marinara:
- 1 tablespoon extra-virgin olive oil
- 3 garlic cloves, minced
- Handful basil leaves
- 1 (28-ounce / 794-g) can chopped tomatoes with juice reserved

Directions:

- Preheat the oven to 350°F (180°C). Line a baking sheet with parchment paper. Heat the olive oil in a nonstick skillet over medium heat until shimmering.
- Add the onion and sauté for 5 minutes or until translucent. Sprinkle with fennel seeds, oregano, red pepper flakes, and garlic powder, then cook for 1 minute or until aromatic.
- Pour the sautéed mixture in a food processor and add the beans and bread crumbs. Sprinkle with ground black pepper, then pulse to combine well and the mixture holds together.
- Shape the mixture into balls with a 2-ounce (57-g) cookie scoop, then arrange the balls on the baking sheet.
- Bake in the preheated oven for 30 minutes or until lightly browned. Flip the balls halfway through the cooking time.
- While baking the bean balls, heat the olive oil in a saucepan over medium-high heat until shimmering. Add the garlic and basil and sauté for 2 minutes or until fragrant.
- Fold in the tomatoes and juice. Bring to a boil. Reduce the heat to low. Put the lid on and simmer for 15 minutes.
- Transfer the bean balls on a large plate and baste with marinara before serving.

Chapter 4 - Side and Salad Recipes

41) Veggie ChimiSalad

Preparation Time: 10 minutes

Cooking Time: 25 minutes

Servings: 4

Nutrition: Calories 231 Fat 20.1 g Carbs 20.1 g Protein 4.6 g

Ingredients:
- Roasted vegetables:
- 1 large sweet potato (chopped
- 6 red potatoes, quartered
- 2 whole carrots, chopped
- 2 tablespoons melted coconut oil
- 2 teaspoons curry powder
- 1 cup chopped broccolini
- 2 cups red cabbage, chopped
- 1 medium red bell pepper, sliced
- Chimichurri:
- 5 cloves garlic, chopped
- 1 medium serrano pepper
- 1 cup packed cilantro
- 1 cup parsley
- 3 tablespoons ripe avocado
- 3 tablespoons lime juice
- 1 tablespoon maple syrup
- Water to thin
- Salad:
- 4 cups hearty greens
- 1 medium ripe avocado, chopped
- 3 tablespoons hemp seeds
- Fresh herbs
- 5 medium radishes, sliced
- ¼ cup macadamia nut cheese

Directions:
- Preheat your oven to 400 degrees F.
- In a suitable bowl, toss all the vegetables for roasting with curry powder and oil.
- Divide these vegetables into two roasting pans.
- Bake the vegetables for 25 minutes in the oven.
- Meanwhile, in a blender, blend all chimichurri sauce ingredients until smooth.
- In a salad bowl, toss in all the roasted vegetables, chimichurri sauce and salad ingredients.
- Mix them well then refrigerate to chill.
- Serve.

42) Exotic Quinoa Bowl

Preparation Time: 15 minutes

Cooking Time: 15 minutes

Servings: 4

Nutrition: Calories: 669 Fat: 40g Protein: 17g Carbs: 69g

Ingredients:
- 1½ cups quinoa
- 2 cucumbers, seeded and diced
- 1 small red onion, diced
- 1 large tomato, diced
- 1 handful fresh flat-leaf parsley, chopped
- ½ cup extra-virgin olive oil
- ¼ cup red wine vinegar
- Juice of 1 lemon
- ¾ teaspoon freshly ground black pepper
- 4 heads endive, trimmed and separated into spears
- 1 avocado, pitted, peeled, and diced

Directions:
- In a saucepan, prepare the quinoa according to package directions. Rinse the quinoa under cold running water and drain very well. Transfer to a large bowl. Add the cucumbers, red onion, tomato, and parsley.
- In a small bowl, whisk together the olive oil, vinegar, lemon juice, and pepper. Pour the dressing over the quinoa mixture and toss to coat. Spoon the mixture onto the endive spears and top with the avocado.

43) Linguini with Peas and Parmigiano Reggiano

Preparation Time: 10 minutes

Cooking Time: 10 minutes

Servings: 4

Nutrition: Calories: 480 Protein: 20 g Fat: 11 g Carbs: 73 g

Ingredients:
- 2 eggs
- 1 cup frozen peas
- ½ cup Parmigiano-Reggiano cheese, grated
- 12 ounces linguini
- 1 Tbsp olive oil
- 1 onion, sliced
- Pepper, to taste

Directions:
- In a bowl, combine the zucchini noodles with pepper and the olive oil and toss well. Prepare linguini according to the package. Whisk eggs and mix in cheese.
- Sauté onion in olive oil, then stir in peas. Add pasta to pan. Add egg mixture to the pasta and cook for another 2 min. Season with pepper. Serve hot.

44) Noodles Salad with Peanut Butter Cream

Preparation Time: 10 minutes

Cooking Time: 0 minutes

Servings: 04

Nutrition: Calories 361 Fat 16.3 g Carbs 29.3 g Protein 3.3 g

Ingredients:
- Salad:
- 6 ounces vermicelli noodles, boiled
- 2 medium whole carrots, ribboned
- 2 stalks green onions, chopped
- ¼ cup cilantro, chopped
- 2 tablespoons mint, chopped
- 1 cup packed spinach, chopped
- 1 cup red cabbage, sliced
- 1 medium red bell pepper, sliced
- Dressing:
- ⅓ cup creamy peanut butter
- 3 tablespoons tamari
- 3 tablespoons maple syrup
- 1 teaspoon chili garlic sauce
- 1 medium lime, juiced
- ¼ cup water

Directions:
- Combine all the dressing ingredients in a small bowl.
- In a salad bowl, toss in the noodles, salad, and dressing.
- Mix them well then refrigerate to chill.
- Serve.

45) Delicious Potato Salad with Mustard

Preparation Time: 15 minutes

Cooking Time: 10 minutes

Servings: 4-6

Nutrition: Calories: 140 Carbs: 1g Fat: 15g Protein: 1g

Ingredients:
- ¼ cup extra-virgin olive oil
- ½ teaspoon pepper
- 1 garlic clove, peeled and threaded on skewer
- 1 small shallot, minced
- 1 tablespoon minced fresh chervil
- 1 tablespoon minced fresh chives
- 1 tablespoon minced fresh parsley
- 1 teaspoon minced fresh tarragon
- 1½ tablespoons white wine vinegar or Champagne vinegar
- 2 pounds small red potatoes, unpeeled, sliced ¼ inch thick
- 2 teaspoons Dijon mustard

Directions:
- Place potatoes in a big saucepan, put in water to cover by 1 inch, and bring to boil on high heat. Put in salt, decrease the heat to simmer, and cook until potatoes are soft and paring knife can be slipped in and out of potatoes with little resistance, about 6 minutes.
- While potatoes are cooking, lower skewered garlic into simmering water and blanch for 45 seconds. Run garlic under cold running water, then remove from skewer and mince.
- Reserve ¼ cup cooking water, then drain potatoes and lay out on tight one layer in rimmed baking sheet.
- Beat oil, minced garlic, vinegar, mustard, pepper, and reserved potato cooking water together in a container, then drizzle over potatoes. Let potatoes sit until flavors blend, about 10 minutes.
- Move potatoes to big container. Mix shallot and herbs in a small-sized container, then drizzle over potatoes and gently toss to coat using rubber spatula. Serve.

46) Easy Creamy Kernel

Preparation Time: 5minutes

Cooking Time:

Servings: 2

Nutrition: Carbs: 44.5g Protein: 11.5g Fats: 11.4g Calories: 306

Ingredients:
- Frozen peas: 1 cup can washed and drained
- Corn kernel: 2 cups can
- Sesame seeds: 2 tbsp
- Pepper: as per your taste
- Cashew cream: ½ cup

Directions:
- Combine all the ingredients
- Serve as the side dish

47) Green Bean with Walnut Mix

Preparation Time: 15 minutes

Cooking Time: 15 minutes

Servings: 6-8

Nutrition: Calories: 145 Carbs: 0g Fat: 8g Protein: 0g

Ingredients:
- ¼ cup walnuts
- ½ cup extra-virgin olive oil
- 1 scallion, sliced thin
- 2 garlic cloves, unpeeled
- 2 pounds green beans, trimmed
- 2½ cups fresh cilantro leaves and stems, tough stem ends trimmed (about 2 bunches)
- 4 teaspoons lemon juice

Directions:
- Cook walnuts and garlic in 8-inch frying pan on moderate heat, stirring frequently, until toasted and aromatic, 5 to 7 minutes; move to a container. Let garlic cool slightly, then peel and approximately chop.
- Process walnuts, garlic, cilantro, oil, lemon juice, scallion, and 1/8 teaspoon pepper using a food processor until smooth, about 1 minute, scraping down sides of the container as required; move to big container.
- Bring 4 quarts water to boil in large pot on high heat. In the meantime, fill big container halfway with ice and water.
- Put in green beans to boiling water and cook until crisp-tender, 3 to 5 minutes. Drain green beans, move to ice water, and allow to sit until chilled, approximately two minutes.
- Move green beans to a container with cilantro sauce and gently toss until coated. Sprinkle with pepper to taste. Serve.

48) Old School Panzanella

Preparation Time: 15 minutes

Cooking Time: 20 minutes

Servings: 6

Nutrition: Calories: 294 Carbs: 32g Fat: 15g Protein: 9g

Ingredients:
- 1 (15-ounce) can cannellini beans, rinsed
- 1 small red onion, halved and sliced thin
- 1½ pounds ripe tomatoes, cored and chopped, seeds and juice reserved
- 12 ounces rustic Italian bread, cut into 1-inch pieces (4 cups)
- 2 ounces Parmesan cheese, shaved
- 2 tablespoons minced fresh oregano
- 3 ounces (3 cups) baby arugula
- 3 tablespoons chopped fresh basil
- 3 tablespoons red wine vinegar
- 5 tablespoons extra-virgin olive oil

Directions:
- Place the oven rack in the center of the oven and pre-heat your oven to 350 degrees. Toss bread pieces with 1 tablespoon oil and sprinkle with pepper.
- Arrange bread in one layer in rimmed baking sheet and bake, stirring intermittently, until light golden brown, fifteen to twenty minutes. Allow it to cool to room temperature.
- Beat vinegar in a big container. Whisking continuously, slowly drizzle in remaining ¼ cup oil.
- Put in tomatoes with their seeds and juice, beans, onion, 1½ tablespoons basil, and 1 tablespoon oregano, toss to coat, and allow to sit for 20 minutes.
- Put in cooled croutons, arugula, remaining 1½ tablespoons basil, and remaining 1 tablespoon oregano and gently toss to combine.
- Sprinkle with pepper to taste. Move salad to serving platter and drizzle with Parmesan. Serve.

49) Vegan Chorizo Salad with Red Wine Vinegar

Preparation Time: 5 minutes

Cooking Time: 5 minutes

Servings: 4

Nutrition: Calories 138, Fat 8.95g, Carbs 5.63g, Protein 7.12g

Ingredients:
- 2 ½ tbsp olive oil
- 4 soy chorizo, chopped
- 2 tsp red wine vinegar
- 1 small red onion, finely chopped
- 2 ½ cups cherry tomatoes, halved
- 2 tbsp chopped cilantro
- Freshly ground black pepper to taste
- 3 tbsp sliced black olives to garnish

Directions:
- Over medium fire, heat half tablespoon of olive oil in a skillet and fry soy chorizo until golden. Turn heat off.
- In a salad bowl, whisk remaining olive oil and vinegar. Add onion, cilantro, tomatoes, and soy chorizo. Mix with dressing and season with black pepper.
- Garnish with olives and serve.

50) Juicy Smoked Apple Salad

Preparation Time: 15 minutes

Cooking Time: 0 minutes

Servings: 4-6

Nutrition: Calories: 157 Carbs: 12g Fat: 13g Protein: 1g

Ingredients:
- ¼ cup extra-virgin olive oil
- 1 fennel bulb, stalks discarded, bulb halved, cored, and sliced thin
- 1 small shallot, minced
- 1 tablespoon whole-grain mustard
- 2 Granny Smith apples, peeled, cored, and cut into 3-inch-long matchsticks
- 2 teaspoons minced fresh tarragon
- 3 tablespoons lemon juice
- 5 ounces (5 cups) watercress
- 6 ounces smoked mackerel, skin and pin bones removed, flaked
- Pepper

Directions:
- Beat lemon juice, mustard, shallot, 1 teaspoon tarragon, and ¼ teaspoon pepper together in a big container.
- Whisking continuously, slowly drizzle in oil. Put in watercress, apples, and fennel and gently toss to coat. Sprinkle with pepper to taste.
- Divide salad among plates and top with flaked mackerel. Sprinkle any remaining dressing over mackerel and drizzle with remaining 1 teaspoon tarragon. Serve instantly.

51) Kalamata Pepper Salad with Pine Nuts

Preparation Time: 10 minutes

Cooking Time: 20 minutes

Servings: 4

Nutrition: Calories 163, Fat 13.3g, Carbs 6.53g, Protein 3.37g

Ingredients:
- 8 large red bell peppers, deseeded and cut in wedges
- ½ tsp erythritol
- 2 ½ tbsp olive oil
- 1/3 cup arugula
- 1 tbsp mint leaves
- 1/3 cup pitted Kalamata olives
- 3 tbsp chopped almonds
- ½ tbsp balsamic vinegar
- Crumbled feta cheese for topping
- Toasted pine nuts for topping

Directions:
- Preheat oven to 400o F.
- Pour bell peppers on a roasting pan; season with erythritol and drizzle with half of olive oil. Roast in oven until slightly charred, 20 minutes. Remove from oven and set aside.
- Arrange arugula in a salad bowl, scatter bell peppers on top, mint leaves, olives, almonds, and drizzle with balsamic vinegar and remaining olive oil. Season with black pepper.
- Toss; top with feta cheese and pine nuts and serve.

52) Spiced Carrot Bowl

Preparation Time: 15 minutes

Cooking Time: 0 minutes

Servings: 4-6

Nutrition: Calories: 84 Carbs: 13g Fat: 4g Protein: 1g

Ingredients:
- 1/8 teaspoon cayenne pepper
- 1/8 teaspoon ground cinnamon
- ¾ teaspoon ground cumin
- 1-pound carrots, peeled and shredded
- 1 tablespoon lemon juice
- 1 teaspoon honey
- 2 oranges
- 3 tablespoons extra-virgin olive oil
- 3 tablespoons minced fresh cilantro

Directions:
- Cut away peel and pith from oranges. Holding fruit over bowl, use paring knife to slice between membranes to release segments.
- Cut segments in half crosswise and allow to drain in fine-mesh strainer set over big container, reserving juice.
- Beat lemon juice, honey, cumin, cayenne, cinnamon into reserved orange juice.
- Put in drained oranges and carrots and gently toss to coat. Allow to sit until liquid starts to pool in bottom of bowl, 3 to 5 minutes.
- Drain salad in fine-mesh strainer and return to now-empty bowl. Mix in cilantro and oil and sprinkle with pepper to taste. Serve.

53) Double Green Juicy Salad

Preparation Time: 10 minutes

Cooking Time: 15 minutes

Servings: 4

Nutrition: Calories 237, Fat 19.57g, Carbs 5.9g, Protein 12.75g

Ingredients:
- 1 (7 ozblock extra firm tofu
- 2 tbsp olive oil
- 2 tbsp butter
- 1 cup asparagus, trimmed and halved
- 1 cup green beans, trimmed
- 2 tbsp chopped dulse
- Freshly ground black pepper to taste
- ½ lemon, juiced
- 4 tbsp chopped walnuts

Directions:
- Place tofu in between two paper towels and allow soaking for 5 minutes. After, remove towels and chop into small cubes.
- Heat olive oil in a skillet and fry tofu until golden, 10 minutes. Remove onto a paper towel-lined plate and set aside.
- Melt butter in skillet and sauté asparagus
- And green beans until softened, 5 minutes. Add dulse, season with black pepper, and Cooking Time: until softened. Mix in tofu and stir-fry for 5 minutes.
- Plate, drizzle with lemon juice, and scatter walnuts on top.
- Serve warm.

54) Lemony Orange Fennel Salad

Preparation Time: 15 minutes

Cooking Time: 0 minutes

Servings: 4-6

Nutrition: Calories: 180 **Carbs:** 21g **Fat:** 11g **Protein:** 3g

Ingredients:
- ¼ cup coarsely chopped fresh mint
- ¼ cup extra-virgin olive oil
- ½ cup pitted oil-cured black olives, quartered
- 2 fennel bulbs, stalks discarded, bulbs halved, cored, and sliced thin
- 2 tablespoons lemon juice
- 4 blood oranges
- Pepper

Directions:
- Cut away peel and pith from oranges. Quarter oranges, then slice crosswise into ¼-inch-thick pieces. Mix oranges, fennel, olives, and mint in a big container.
- Beat lemon juice, and 1/8 teaspoon pepper together in a small-sized container. Whisking continuously, slowly drizzle in oil.
- Sprinkle dressing over salad and gently toss to coat. Sprinkle with pepper to taste. Serve.

55) Asian Goji Salad

Preparation Time: 10 minutes

Cooking Time: 2 minutes

Servings: 4

Nutrition: Calories 203, **Fat** 15.28g, **Carbs** 9.64g, **Protein** 6.67g, **Protein** 2.54g

Ingredients:
- 1 small head cauliflower, cut into florets
- 8 sun-dried tomatoes in olive oil, drained
- 12 pitted green olives, roughly chopped
- 1 lemon, zested and juiced
- 3 tbsp chopped green onions
- A handful chopped almonds
- ¼ cup goji berries
- 1 tbsp sesame oil
- ½ cup watercress
- 3 tbsp chopped parsley
- Freshly ground black pepper to taste
- Lemon wedges to garnish

Directions:
- Pour cauliflower into a large safe-microwave bowl, sprinkle with some water, and steam in microwave for 1 to 2 minutes or until softened.
- In a large salad bowl, combine cauliflower, tomatoes, olives, lemon zest and juice, green onions, almonds, goji berries, sesame oil, watercress, and parsley. Season with black pepper, and mix well.
- Serve with lemon wedges.

56) Cheesy Asparagus Pesto Salad

Preparation Time: 15 minutes

Cooking Time: 0 minutes

Servings: 4-6

Nutrition: Calories: 220 **Carbs:** 40g **Fat:** 5g **Protein:** 6g

Ingredients:
Pesto:
- ¼ cup fresh basil leaves
- ¼ cup grated Pecorino Romano cheese
- ½ cup extra-virgin olive oil
- 1 garlic clove, minced
- 1 teaspoon grated lemon zest plus 2 teaspoons juice
- 2 cups fresh mint leaves
- Pepper

Salad:
- ¾ cup hazelnuts, toasted, skinned, and chopped
- 2 oranges
- 2 pounds asparagus, trimmed
- 4 ounces feta cheese, crumbled (1 cup)
- Pepper

Directions:
- For the Pesto, process mint, basil, Pecorino, lemon zest and juice, garlic, and ¾ teaspoon salt using a food processor until finely chopped, approximately half a minute, scraping down sides of the container as required. Move to big container. Mix in oil and sprinkle with pepper to taste.
- For the Salad, chop asparagus tips from stalks into ¾-inch-long pieces. Cut asparagus stalks 1/8 inch thick on bias into approximate 2-inch lengths.
- Cut away the peel and pith from oranges. Holding fruit over bowl, use paring knife to cut between membranes to release segments.
- Put in asparagus tips and stalks, orange segments, feta, and hazelnuts to pesto and toss to combine. Sprinkle with pepper to taste. Serve.

57) Ricotta Seed Salad

Preparation Time: 15 minutes

Cooking Time:

Servings: 4

Nutrition: Calories 397, **Fat** 3.87g, **Carbs** 8.4g, **Protein** 8.93g

Ingredients:
- 2 tbsp olive oil
- 1 tbsp white wine vinegar
- 2 tbsp chia seeds
- Freshly ground black pepper to taste
- 2 cups broccoli slaw
- 1 cup chopped kelp, thoroughly washed and steamed
- 1/3 cup chopped pecans
- 1/3 cup pumpkin seeds
- 1/3 cup blueberries
- 2/3 cup ricotta cheese

Directions:
- In a small bowl, whisk olive oil, white wine vinegar, chia seeds, and black pepper. Set aside.
- In a large salad bowl, combine the broccoli slaw, kelp, pecans, pumpkin seeds, blueberries, and ricotta cheese.
- Drizzle dressing on top, toss, and serve.

58) Veggie Almond Chermoula Bowl

Preparation Time: 15 minutes

Cooking Time: 22 minutes

Servings: 4-6

Nutrition: Calories: 450 Carbs: 77g Fat: 7g Protein: 20g

Ingredients:

Salad:
- ½ cup raisins
- ½ red onion, sliced ¼ inch thick
- 1 cup shredded carrot
- 1 head cauliflower (2 pounds), cored and cut into 2-inch florets
- 2 tablespoons chopped fresh cilantro
- 2 tablespoons extra-virgin olive oil
- 2 tablespoons sliced almonds, toasted
- Pepper

Chermoula:
- 1/8 teaspoon cayenne pepper
- ¼ cup extra-virgin olive oil
- ½ teaspoon ground cumin
- ½ teaspoon paprika
- ¾ cup fresh cilantro leaves
- 2 tablespoons lemon juice
- 4 garlic cloves, minced

Directions:

- For the salad, place oven rack to lowest position and pre-heat your oven to 475 degrees. Toss cauliflower with oil and sprinkle with pepper.
- Arrange cauliflower in one layer in parchment paper–lined rimmed baking sheet. Cover tightly with aluminum foil and roast till they become tender, 5 to 7 minutes.
- Remove foil and spread onion evenly in sheet. Roast until vegetables are tender, cauliflower becomes deeply golden brown, and onion slices are charred at edges, 10 to 15 minutes, stirring halfway through roasting. Allow it to cool slightly, approximately five minutes.
- For the chermoula, process all ingredients using a food processor until smooth, about 1 minute, scraping down sides of the container as required. Move to big container.
- Gently toss cauliflower-onion mixture, carrot, raisins, and cilantro with chermoula until coated. Move to serving platter and drizzle with almonds. Serve warm or at room temperature.

59) Baked Asparagus Maple Salad

Preparation Time: 10 minutes

Cooking Time: 20 minutes

Servings: 4

Nutrition: Calories 146, Fat 12.87g, Carbs 5.07g, Protein 4.44g

Ingredients:

- 1 lb asparagus, trimmed and halved
- 2 tbsp olive oil
- ½ tsp dried basil
- ½ tsp dried oregano
- Freshly ground black pepper to taste
- ½ tsp hemp seeds
- 1 tbsp maple (sugar-free syrup
- ½ cup arugula
- 4 tbsp crumbled feta cheese
- 2 tbsp hazelnuts
- 1 lemon, cut into wedges

Directions:

- Preheat oven to 350oF.
- Pour asparagus on a baking tray, drizzle with olive oil, basil, oregano, black pepper, and hemp seeds. Mix with your hands and roast in oven for 15 minutes.
- Remove, drizzle with maple syrup, and continue cooking until slightly charred, 5 minutes.
- Spread arugula in a salad bowl and top with asparagus. Scatter with feta cheese, hazelnuts, and serve with lemon wedges.

60) Cherry Kalamata Salad with Oregano

Preparation Time: 15 minutes

Cooking Time: 10 minutes

Servings: 4-6

Nutrition: Calories: 110 Carbs: 20g Fat: 4g Protein: 1g

Ingredients:

- ½ cup pitted kalamata olives, chopped
- ½ teaspoon sugar
- 1 shallot, minced
- 1 small cucumber, peeled, halved along the length, seeded, and cut into ½-inch pieces
- 1 tablespoon red wine vinegar
- 1½ pounds cherry tomatoes, quartered
- 2 garlic cloves, minced
- 2 tablespoons extra-virgin olive oil
- 2 teaspoons minced fresh oregano
- 3 tablespoons chopped fresh parsley
- 4 ounces feta cheese, crumbled (1 cup)
- Pepper

Directions:

- Toss tomatoes with sugar and ¼ teaspoon salt in a container and allow to sit for 30 minutes.
- Move tomatoes to salad spinner and spin until seeds and excess liquid have been removed, 45 to 60 seconds, stopping to redistribute tomatoes several times during spinning.
- Put in tomatoes, cucumber, olives, feta, and parsley to big container; set aside.
- Strain ½ cup tomato liquid through fine-mesh strainer into liquid measuring cup; discard remaining liquid.
- Bring tomato liquid, shallot, vinegar, garlic, and oregano to simmer in small saucepan on moderate heat and cook until reduced to 3 tablespoons, 6 to 8 minutes.
- Move to small-sized container and allow to cool to room temperature, approximately five minutes. Whisking continuously, slowly drizzle in oil.
- Sprinkle dressing over salad and gently toss to coat. Sprinkle with pepper to taste. Serve.

Chapter 5 - Main Recipes

61) Zucchini Rice with Chicken Chunks

Preparation Time: 10 minutes

Cooking Time: 14 minutes

Servings: 4

Nutrition: Calories 500 Fat 16.5 g Carbs 48 g Protein 38.7 g

Ingredients:
- 3 chicken breasts, skinless, boneless, and cut into chunks
- 1/4 fresh parsley, chopped
- 1 zucchini, sliced
- 2 bell peppers, chopped
- 1 cup rice, rinsed and drained
- 1 1/2 cup chicken broth
- 1 tbsp oregano
- 3 tbsp fresh lemon juice
- 1 tbsp garlic, minced
- 1 onion, diced
- 2 tbsp olive oil
- Pepper

Directions:
- Add oil into the inner pot of instant pot and set the pot on sauté mode. Add onion and chicken and cook for 5 minutes. Add rice, oregano, lemon juice, garlic, broth, pepper, and stir everything well.
- Seal pot with lid and cook on high for 4 minutes. Once done, release pressure using quick release. Remove lid. Add parsley, zucchini, and bell peppers and stir well.
- Seal pot again with lid and select manual and set timer for 5 minutes. Release pressure using quick release. Remove lid. Stir well and serve.

62) Smoked Baby Spinach Stew

Preparation Time: 10 minutes

Cooking Time: 25 minutes

Servings: 4

Nutrition: Calories 369 Fat 9.7g Carbs 67.9g Protein 18g

Ingredients:
- 1 splash olive oil
- 1 small onion, chopped
- 2 cloves garlic
- 5g cumin powder
- 5g smoked paprika
- ¼ teaspoon chili powder
- 235ml water
- 670g can diced tomatoes
- 165g cooked chickpeas (or can chickpeas
- 60g baby spinach
- A handful of chopped coriander, to garnish
- 20g slivered almonds, to garnish
- 4 slices toasted whole-grain bread, to serve

Directions:
- Heat olive oil in a saucepan over medium-high heat.
- Add onion and Cooking Time: until browned, for 7-8 minutes.
- Add garlic, cumin, paprika, and chili powder.
- Cooking Time: 1 minute.
- Add water and scrape any browned bits.
- Add the tomatoes and chickpeas. Season to taste and reduce heat.
- Simmer the soup for 10 minutes.
- Stir in spinach and Cooking Time: 2 minutes.
- Ladle soup in a bowl. Sprinkle with cilantro and almonds.
- Serve with toasted bread slices.

63) Green Chilis Chicken Breast

Preparation Time: 10 minutes

Cooking Time: 10 minutes

Servings: 3

Nutrition: Calories 237 Fat 8 g Carbs 10.8 g Protein 30.5 g

Ingredients:
- 2 chicken breasts, skinless and boneless
- 1 tbsp chili powder
- 1/2 tsp ground cumin
- 1/2 tsp garlic powder
- 1/4 tsp onion powder
- 1/2 tsp paprika
- 4 oz can green chilis, diced
- 1/4 cup chicken broth
- 14 oz can tomato, diced
- Pepper

Directions:
- Add all ingredients except chicken into the instant pot and stir well. Add chicken and stir. Seal pot with lid and cook on high for 10 minutes.
- Once done, allow to release pressure naturally for 5 minutes then release remaining using quick release. Remove lid.
- Remove chicken from pot and shred using a fork. Return shredded chicken to the pot and stir well. Serve and enjoy.

64) Chicken Breast with Italian Seasoning

Preparation Time: 10 minutes

Cooking Time: 12 minutes

Servings: 8

Nutrition: Calories 502 Fat 20 g Carbs 7.8 g Protein 66.8 g

Ingredients:
- 4 lb. chicken breasts, skinless and boneless
- 1 tbsp garlic powder
- 2 tbsp dried Italian herb mix
- 2 tbsp olive oil
- 1/4 cup chicken stock
- Pepper

Directions:
- Coat chicken with oil and season with dried herb, garlic powder, pepper. Place chicken into the instant pot. Pour stock over the chicken. Seal pot with a lid and select manual and set timer for 12 minutes.
- Once done, allow to release pressure naturally for 5 minutes then release remaining using quick release. Remove lid. Shred chicken using a fork and serve.

65) Veggie Ragù Noodles

Preparation Time: 10 minutes

Cooking Time: 15 minutes (plus 25 for lentils

Servings: 4

Nutrition: Calories 353 Fat 0.9g Carbs 74g Protein 17.7g

Ingredients:
- Bolognese:
- 100g red lentils
- 1 bay leaf
- Splash of olive oil
- 1 small onion, diced
- 1 large stalk celery, sliced
- 3 cloves garlic, minced
- 230ml tomato sauce or fresh pureed tomatoes
- 60ml red wine or vegetable stock (if you do not like wine
- 1 tablespoon fresh basil, chopped
- Pepper, to taste
- Soba noodles:
- 280g soba noodles

Directions:
- Cooking Time: the lentils; place lentils and bay leaf in a saucepan.
- Cover with water, so the water is 2-inches above the lentils.
- Bring to a boil over medium-high heat.
- Reduce heat and simmer the lentils for 25 minutes.
- Drain the lentils and discard the bay leaf.
- Heat a splash of olive oil in a saucepan.
- Add onion, and Cooking Time: 6 minutes.
- Add celery and Cooking Time: 2 minutes.
- Add garlic and Cooking Time: 2 minutes.
- Add the tomatoes and wine. Simmer the mixture for 5 minutes.
- Stir in the lentils and simmer 2 minutes.
- Remove the Bolognese from the heat and stir in basil.
- In the meantime, Cooking Time: the soba noodles according to package directions.
- Serve noodles with lentils Bolognese.

66) Quinoa Chicken with Olives and Grrek Seasoning

Preparation Time: 10 minutes

Cooking Time: 6 minutes

Servings: 4

Nutrition: Calories 566 Fat 16.4 g Carbs 57.4 g Protein 46.8 g

Ingredients:
- 1 lb. chicken breasts, skinless, boneless, and cut into chunks
- 14 oz can chickpeas, drained and rinsed
- 1 cup olives, pitted and sliced
- 1 cup cherry tomatoes, halved
- 1 cucumber, sliced
- 2 tsp Greek seasoning
- 1 1/2 cups chicken broth
- 1 cup quinoa, rinsed and drained
- Pepper

Directions:
- Add broth and quinoa into the instant pot and stir well. Season chicken with Greek seasoning, pepper and place into the instant pot.
- Seal pot with lid and cook on high for 6 minutes. Once done, release pressure using quick release. Remove lid. Stir quinoa and chicken mixture well.
- Add remaining ingredients and stir everything well. Serve immediately and enjoy it.

67) Red Quinoa Burgers with Thaini Guacamole

Preparation Time: 10 minutes

Cooking Time: 50 minutes

Servings: 4

Nutrition: Calories 343 Fat 16.6g Total Carbs 49.1g Protein 15g

Ingredients:
- Patties:
- 2 large beets, peeled, cubed
- 1 red onion, cut into chunks
- 115g red kidney beans
- 85g red cooked quinoa
- 2 cloves garlic, minced
- 30g almond meal
- 20g ground flax
- 10ml lemon juice
- ½ teaspoon ground cumin
- ½ teaspoon red pepper flakes
- 4 whole-meal burger buns
- Tahini Guacamole:
- 1 avocado, pitted, peeled
- 45ml lime juice
- 30g tahini sauce
- 5g chopped coriander

Directions:
- Preheat oven to 190C/375F.
- Toss beet and onion with a splash of olive oil.
- Bake the beets for 30 minutes.
- Transfer the beets and onion into a food blender.
- Add the beans and blend until coarse. You do not want a completely smooth mixture.
- Stir in quinoa, garlic, almond meal, flax seeds, lemon juice, cumin, and red pepper flakes.
- Shape the mixture into four patties.
- Transfer the patties to a baking sheet, lined with parchment paper.
- Bake the patties 20 minutes, flipping halfway through.
- In the meantime, make the tahini guac; mash the avocado with lime juice in a bowl.
- Stir in tahini and coriander. Season to taste.
- To serve; place the patty in the bun, top with guacamole and serve.

68) Rice and Beans with Red Bell pepper

Preparation Time: 10 minutes

Cooking Time: 1 hour 10 minutes

Servings: 6

Nutrition: Calories 469 Fat 6g Carbs 87.5g Protein 21.1g

Ingredients:
- 450g dry red kidney beans, soaked overnight
- 15ml olive oil
- 1 onion, diced
- 1 red bell pepper, seeded, diced
- 1 large stalk celery, sliced
- 4 cloves garlic, minced
- 15ml hot sauce
- 5g paprika
- 2g dried thyme
- 2 g parsley, chopped
- 2 bay leaves
- 900ml vegetable stock
- 280g brown rice
- Pepper, to taste

Directions:
- Drain the beans and place aside.
- Heat olive oil in a saucepot.
- Add onion and bell pepper. Cooking Time: 6 minutes.
- Add celery and Cooking Time: 3 minutes.
- Add garlic, hot sauce, paprika, and thyme. Cooking Time: 1 minute.
- Add the drained beans, bay leaves, and vegetable stock.
- Bring to a boil, and reduce heat.
- Simmer the beans for 1 hour 15 minutes or until tender.
- In the meantime, place rice in a small saucepot. Cover the rice with 4cm water.
- Season to taste and Cooking Time: the rice until tender, for 25 minutes.
- To serve; transfer ¼ of the beans into a food processor. Process until smooth.
- Combine the processed beans with the remaining beans and ladle into a bowl.
- Add rice and sprinkle with parsley before serving.

69) Baked Sole with Pistachos

Preparation Time: 5 minutes

Cooking Time: 10 minutes

Servings: 2

Nutrition: 166 Calories 6g Fat 2g Carbs 6g Protein

Ingredients:
- 4 (5 ounces) boneless sole fillets
- ½ cup pistachios, finely chopped
- Juice of 1 lemon
- teaspoon extra virgin olive oil

Directions:
- Pre-heat your oven to 350 degrees Fahrenheit
- Wrap baking sheet using parchment paper and keep it on the side
- Pat fish dry with kitchen towels and lightly season with salt and pepper
- Take a small bowl and stir in pistachios
- Place sol on the prepped sheet and press 2 tablespoons of pistachio mixture on top of each fillet
- Rub the fish with lemon juice and olive oil
- Bake for 10 minutes until the top is golden and fish flakes with a fork

70) Quinoa with Avocado and Pepper Mix

Preparation Time: 15 minutes

Cooking Time: 1 hour 5 minutes

Servings: 4

Nutrition: Calories 456 Total Fat 15.4g Carbs 71.1g Protein 8g

Ingredients:
- 160g quinoa
- 460ml vegetable stock
- 2 red bell peppers, cut in half, seeds and membrane removed
- 2 yellow bell peppers, cut in half, seeds, and membrane removed
- 120g salsa
- 15g nutritional yeast
- 10g chili powder
- 5g cumin powder
- 425g can black beans, rinsed, drained
- 160g fresh corn kernels
- Pepper, to taste
- 1 small avocado, sliced
- 15g chopped cilantro

Directions:
- Preheat oven to 190C/375F.
- Brush the baking sheet with some cooking oil.
- Combine quinoa and vegetable stock in a saucepan. Bring to a boil.
- Reduce heat and simmer 20 minutes.
- Transfer the quinoa to a large bowl.
- Stir in salsa, nutritional yeast, chili powder, cumin powder, black beans, and corn. Season to taste with pepper.
- Stuff the bell pepper halves with prepared mixture.
- Transfer the peppers onto a baking sheet, cover with aluminum foil, and bake for 30 minutes.
- Increase heat to 200C/400F and bake the peppers for an additional 15 minutes.
- Serve warm, topped with avocado slices, and chopped cilantro.

71) Lemony Mussels in Dry Wine Sauce

Preparation Time: 5 minutes

Cooking Time: 10 minutes

Servings: 2

Nutrition: Calories 22, 7 g fat, 1 g fiber, 18 g protein

Ingredients:
- 2 pounds small mussels
- 1 tablespoon extra-virgin olive oil
- 1 cup thinly sliced red onion
- 3 garlic cloves, sliced
- 1 cup dry white wine
- 2 (¼-inch-thick) lemon slices
- ¼ teaspoon freshly ground black pepper
- Fresh lemon wedges, for serving (optional)

Directions:
- In a large colander in the sink, run cold water over the mussels (but don't let the mussels sit in standing water).
- All the shells should be closed tight; discard any shells that are a little bit open or any shells that are cracked. Leave the mussels in the colander until you're ready to use them.
- In a large skillet over medium-high heat, heat the oil. Add the onion and cook for 4 minutes, stirring occasionally.
- Add the garlic and cook for 1 minute, stirring constantly. Add the wine, lemon slices, pepper, and bring to a simmer. Cook for 2 minutes.
- Add the mussels and cover. Cook for 3 minutes, or until the mussels open their shells. Gently shake the pan two or three times while they are cooking.
- All the shells should now be wide open. Using a slotted spoon, discard any mussels that are still closed. Spoon the opened mussels into a shallow serving bowl, and pour the broth over the top. Serve with additional fresh lemon slices, if desired.

72) Cold Spinach with Fruit Mix

Preparation Time: 5 minutes

Cooking Time: 0 minute

Servings: 1

Nutrition: Calories 296 Fat 18 g Carbs 27 g Protein 8 g

Ingredients:
- 3 cups baby spinach
- ½ cup strawberries, sliced
- 1 tablespoon white onion, chopped
- 2 tablespoons vinaigrette
- ¼ medium avocado, diced
- 2 tablespoons walnut, toasted

Directions:
- Put the spinach, strawberries and onion in a glass jar with lid.
- Drizzle dressing on top.
- Top with avocado and walnuts.
- Seal the lid and refrigerate until ready to serve.

73) Juiced Shrimp with Herbs

Preparation Time: 20 minutes

Cooking Time: 10 minutes

Servings: 2

Nutrition: Calories 190, 8 g fat, 1 g fiber, 24 g protein

Ingredients:
- 1 large orange
- 3 tablespoons extra-virgin olive oil, divided
- 1 tablespoon chopped fresh Rosemary
- 1 tablespoon chopped fresh thyme
- 3 garlic cloves, minced (about 1½ teaspoons)
- ¼ teaspoon freshly ground black pepper
- 1½ pounds fresh raw shrimp, shells, and tails removed

Directions:
- Zest the entire orange using a citrus grater. In a large zip-top plastic bag, combine the orange zest and 2 tablespoons of oil with the Rosemary, thyme, garlic and pepper
- Add the shrimp, seal the bag, and gently massage the shrimp until all the ingredients are combined and the shrimp is completely covered with the seasonings. Set aside.
- Heat a grill, grill pan, or a large skillet over medium heat. Brush on or swirl in the remaining 1 tablespoon of oil.
- Add half the shrimp, and cook for 4 to 6 minutes, or until the shrimp turn pink and white, flipping halfway through if on the grill or stirring every minute if in a pan. Transfer the shrimp to a large serving bowl.
- Repeat with the remaining shrimp, and add them to the bowl.
- While the shrimp cook, peel the orange and cut the flesh into bite-size pieces. Add to the serving bowl, and toss with the cooked shrimp. Serve immediately or refrigerate and serve cold.

74) Veggie Grill with Herbs and Cider Vinegar

Preparation Time: 15 minutes

Cooking Time: 6 minutes

Servings: 6

Nutrition: Calories 127 Fat 9 g Carbs 11 g Protein 3 g

Ingredients:
- 2 teaspoons cider vinegar
- 1 tablespoon olive oil
- ¼ teaspoon fresh thyme, chopped
- 1 teaspoon fresh parsley, chopped
- ¼ teaspoon fresh rosemary, chopped
- Pepper to taste
- 1 onion, sliced into wedges
- 2 red bell peppers, sliced
- 3 tomatoes, sliced in half
- 6 large mushrooms, stems removed
- 1 eggplant, sliced crosswise
- 3 tablespoons olive oil
- 1 tablespoon cider vinegar

Directions:
- Make the dressing by mixing the vinegar, oil, thyme, parsley, rosemary and pepper.
- In a bowl, mix the onion, red bell pepper, tomatoes, mushrooms and eggplant.
- Toss in remaining olive oil and cider vinegar.
- Grill over medium heat for 3 minutes.
- Turn the vegetables and grill for another 3 minutes.
- Arrange grilled vegetables in a food container.
- Drizzle with the herbed mixture when ready to serve.

75) Cheesy Gnocchi with Shrimp

Preparation Time: 10 minutes

Cooking Time: 20 minutes

Servings: 2

Nutrition: Calories 227, 7 g total fat, 1 g fiber, 20 g protein

Ingredients:
- 1 cup chopped fresh tomato
- 2 tablespoons extra-virgin olive oil
- 2 garlic cloves, minced
- ½ teaspoon freshly ground black pepper
- ¼ teaspoon crushed red pepper
- 1 (12-ounces) jar roasted red peppers
- 1-pound fresh raw shrimp, shells and tails removed
- 1-pound frozen gnocchi (not thawed)
- ½ cup cubed feta cheese
- 1/3 cup fresh torn basil leaves

Directions:
- Preheat the oven to 425°F. In a baking dish, mix the tomatoes, oil, garlic, black pepper, and crushed red pepper. Roast in the oven for 10 minutes.
- Stir in the roasted peppers and shrimp. Roast for 10 more minutes, until the shrimp turn pink and white.
- While the shrimp cooks, cook the gnocchi on the stovetop according to the package directions.
- Drain in a colander and keep warm. Remove the dish from the oven. Mix in the cooked gnocchi, feta, and basil, and serve.

76) Hummus Quinoa with Edamame Bowl

Preparation Time: 10 minutes

Cooking Time: 10 minutes

Servings: 4

Nutrition: Calories 381 Fat 19 g Carbs 43 g Protein 16 g

Ingredients:
- 8 oz. microwavable quinoa
- 2 tablespoons lemon juice
- ½ cup hummus
- Water
- 5 oz. baby kale
- 8 oz. cooked baby beets, sliced
- 1 cup frozen shelled edamame (thawed)
- ¼ cup sunflower seeds, toasted
- 1 avocado, sliced
- 1 cup pecans
- 2 tablespoons flaxseeds

Directions:
- Cooking Time: quinoa according to directions in the packaging.
- Set aside and let cool.
- In a bowl, mix the lemon juice and hummus.
- Add water to achieve desired consistency.
- Divide mixture into 4 condiment containers.
- Cover containers with lids and put in the refrigerator.
- Divide the baby kale into 4 food containers with lids.
- Top with quinoa, beets, edamame and sunflower seeds.
- Store in the refrigerator until ready to serve.
- Before serving add avocado slices and hummus dressing.

77) Fresh Salmon Fillet with Pepper

Preparation Time: 5 minutes

Cooking Time: 2 hours

Servings: 2

Nutrition: Calories 446, 20g fat, 65g protein

Ingredients:
- 2 (6-ounce / 170-g) salmon fillets
- 1 tablespoon olive oil
- 2 cloves garlic, minced
- ½ tablespoon lime juice
- 1 teaspoon finely chopped fresh parsley
- ¼ teaspoon black pepper

Directions:
- Spread a length of foil onto a work surface and place the salmon fillets in the middle.
- Blend olive oil, garlic, lime juice, parsley, and black pepper. Brush the mixture over the fillets. Fold the foil over and crimp the sides to make a packet.
- Place the packet into the slow cooker, cover, and cook on High for 2 hours
- Serve hot.

78) Delicious Puttanesca with Fresh Shrimp

Preparation Time: 5 minutes

Cooking Time: 15 minutes

Servings: 2

Nutrition: Calories 214, 10 g fat, 2 g fiber, 26 g protein

Ingredients:
- 2 tablespoons extra-virgin olive oil
- 3 anchovy fillets, drained and chopped
- 3 garlic cloves, minced
- ½ teaspoon crushed red pepper
- 1 (14.5-ounces) can low-sodium or no-salt-added diced tomatoes, undrained
- 1 (2.25-ounces) can sliced black olives, drained
- 2 tablespoons capers
- 1 tablespoon chopped fresh oregano
- 1-pound fresh raw shrimp, shells and tails removed

Directions:
- In a large skillet over medium heat, heat the oil. Mix in the anchovies, garlic, and crushed red pepper.
- Cook for 3 minutes, stirring frequently and mashing up the anchovies with a wooden spoon until they have melted into the oil.
- Stir in the tomatoes with their juices, olives, capers, and oregano. Turn up the heat to medium-high, and bring to a simmer.
- When the sauce is lightly bubbling, stir in the shrimp. Reduce the heat to medium, and cook the shrimp for 6 to 8 minutes, or until they turn pink and white, stirring occasionally, and serve.

79) Different Spicy Lasagna

Preparation Time: 15 minutes

Cooking Time: 40 minutes

Servings: 4

Nutrition: Calories: 194, **Fat:** 17.4g, **Carbs:** 7g, **Protein:** 7g

Ingredients:
- 2 tbsp butter
- 1 ½ lb ground tempeh
- Salt and ground black pepper to taste
- 1 tsp garlic powder
- 1 tsp onion powder
- 2 tbsp coconut flour
- 1 ½ cup grated mozzarella cheese
- 1/3 cup parmesan cheese
- 2 cups crumbled cottage cheese
- 1 large egg, beaten into a bowl
- 2 cups unsweetened marinara sauce
- 1 tbsp dried Italian mixed herbs
- ¼ tsp red chili flakes
- 4 large yellow squash, sliced
- ¼ cup fresh basil leaves

Directions:
- Preheat the oven to 375 F and grease a baking dish with cooking spray. Set aside.
- Melt the butter in a large skillet over medium heat and Cooking Time: the tempeh until brown, 10 minutes. Set aside to cool.
- In a medium bowl, mix the garlic powder, onion powder, coconut flour, black pepper, mozzarella cheese, half of the parmesan cheese, cottage cheese, and egg. Set aside.
- In another bowl, combine the marinara sauce, mixed herbs, and red chili flakes. Set aside.
- Make a single layer of the squash slices in the baking dish; spread a quarter of the egg mixture on top, a layer of the tempeh, then a quarter of the marinara sauce. Repeat the layering process in the same
- Ingredient proportions and sprinkle the top with the remaining parmesan cheese.
- Bake in the oven until golden brown on top, 30 minutes.
- Remove the dish from the oven, allow cooling for 5 minutes, garnish with the basil leaves, slice and serve.

80) Italian Green Seitan

Preparation Time: 15 minutes

Cooking Time: 18 minutes

Servings: 4

Nutrition: Calories: 582, **Fat:** 49.7g, **Carbs:** 8g, **Protein:** 31g,

Ingredients:
- 1 ½ lb seitan
- 3 tbsp almond flour
- Black pepper to taste
- 2 large zucchinis, cut into 2-inch slices
- 4 tbsp olive oil
- 2 tsp Italian mixed herb blend
- ½ cup vegetable broth

Directions:
- Preheat the oven to 400 F.
- Cut the seitan into strips and set aside.
- In a zipper bag, add the almond flour, salt, and black pepper. Mix and add the seitan slices. Seal the bag and shake to coat the seitan with the seasoning.
- Grease a baking sheet with cooking spray and arrange the zucchinis on the baking sheet. Season with black pepper, and drizzle with 2 tablespoons of olive oil.
- Using tongs, remove the seitan from the almond flour mixture, shake off the excess flour, and put two to three seitan strips on each zucchini.
- Season with the herb blend and drizzle again with olive oil.
- Cooking Time: in the oven for 8 minutes; remove the sheet and carefully pour in the vegetable broth. Bake further for 5 to 10 minutes or until the seitan cooks through.
- Remove from the oven and serve warm with low carb bread.

Chapter 6 -   Soup Recipes

81) Smoked Red Soup

Preparation Time: 10 minutes

Cooking Time: 17 minutes

Servings: 06

Nutrition: Calories 119 Fat 14 g Carbs 19 g Protein 5g

Ingredients:
- 1¼ cups red lentils, rinsed
- 4 cups of water
- ½ cup diced red bell pepper
- 1¼ cups red salsa
- 1 tablespoon chili powder
- 1 tablespoon dried oregano
- 1 teaspoon smoked paprika
- ¼ teaspoon black pepper
- ¾ cup frozen sweet corn
- 2 tablespoons lime juice

Directions:
- In a saucepan, add all the ingredients except the corn.
- Put on saucepan's lid and Cooking Time: for 15 minutes at a simmer.
- Stir in corn and Cooking Time: for another 2 minutes.
- Serve.

82) Lettuce Egg Soup Bowl

Preparation Time: 15 minutes

Cooking Time: 10 minutes

Servings: 2

Nutrition: Calories: 158 Carbs: 6.9g Fats: 7.3g Proteins: 15.4g

Ingredients:
- 32 oz vegetable broth
- 2 eggs
- 1 head romaine lettuce, chopped

Directions:
- Bring the vegetable broth to a boil and reduce the heat. Poach the eggs for 5 minutes in the broth and remove them into 2 bowls.
- Stir in romaine lettuce into the broth and cook for 4 minutes. Dish out in a bowl and serve hot.

83) Cayenne Kale and Mushrooms Soup

Preparation Time: 10 minutes

Cooking Time: 5 hrs. 5 minutes

Servings: 08

Nutrition: Calories 231 Fat 20.1 g Carbs 19,9 g Protein 4.6 g

Ingredients:
- ¼ cup olive oil
- 10 ounces button mushrooms, cleaned, and sliced
- 1½ teaspoons smoked paprika
- 1 pinch ground cayenne pepper
- 1 large onion, diced
- 2 cloves garlic, minced
- 2 pounds russet potatoes, peeled and diced
- 7 cups vegetable broth
- 8 ounces kale, sliced
- ½ teaspoon black pepper

Directions:
- In a pan, heat cooking oil and sauté mushrooms for 12 minutes.
- Season the mushrooms with salt, cayenne pepper, and paprika.
- Add olive oil and onion to a slow cooker.
- Sauté for 5 minutes then toss in rest of the soup ingredients.
- Put on the slow cooker's lid and Cooking Time: for 5 hours on low heat.
- Once done, puree the soup with a hand blender.
- Stir in sautéed mushrooms.
- Serve.

84) Coco Butternut Soup

Preparation Time: 15 minutes

Cooking Time: 1 hour & 35 minutes

Servings: 4

Nutrition: Calories: 149 Carbs: 6.6g Fats: 11.6g Proteins: 5.4g

Ingredients:
- 1 small onion, chopped
- 4 cups chicken broth
- 1 butternut squash
- 3 tablespoons coconut oil
- Nutmeg and pepper, to taste

Directions:
- Put oil and onions in a large pot and add onions. Sauté for about 3 minutes and add chicken broth and butternut squash.
- Simmer for about 1 hour on medium heat and transfer into an immersion blender. Pulse until smooth and season with pepper and nutmeg.
- Return to the pot and cook for about 30 minutes. Dish out and serve hot.

85) Cauliflower Broth with Leek

Preparation Time: 15 minutes

Cooking Time: 1 hour & 31 minutes

Servings: 4

Nutrition: Calories: 185 Carbs: 5.8g Fats: 12.7g Proteins: 10.8g

Ingredients:
- 4 cups chicken broth
- ½ cauliflower head, chopped
- 1 leek, chopped
- Black pepper, to taste

Directions:
- Put the cauliflower, leek and chicken broth into the pot and cook for about 1 hour on medium heat. Transfer into an immersion blender and pulse until smooth.
- Cook on for about 30 minutes on low heat. Season with pepper and serve.

86) Split Veggie Soup

Preparation Time: 10 minutes

Cooking Time: 6 hours

Servings: 12

Nutrition: Calories 361 Fat 16.3 g Carbs 29.3 g Protein 3.3 g

Ingredients:
- 1 cup dried, green split peas
- 2 cups celery, chopped
- 2 cups sliced carrots
- 1½ cups cauliflower, chopped
- 2 ounces dried shiitake mushrooms, chopped
- 9 ounces frozen artichoke hearts
- 11 cups water
- 1 teaspoon garlic powder
- 1½ teaspoon onion powder
- ½ teaspoon black pepper
- 1 tablespoon parsley
- ½ teaspoon ginger
- ½ teaspoon ground mustard seed
- ½ tablespoon brown rice vinegar

Directions:
- Add all the ingredients to a slow cooker.
- Put on the slow cooker's lid and Cooking
- Time: for 6 hours on low heat.
- Once done, garnish as desired.
- Serve warm.

87) Minestrone Bean Soup

Preparation Time: 10 minutes

Cooking Time: 2hrs 2 minutes

Servings: 4

Nutrition: Calories 205 Fat 19.7 g Carbs 26.1 g Protein 5.2 g

Ingredients:
- ½ sweet onion, chopped
- 4 garlic cloves, chopped
- 1 small head broccoli, chopped
- 2 stalks celery, chopped
- 1 cup green peas
- 3 green onions, chopped
- 2¾ cups vegetable broth
- 4 cups leafy greens
- 1 (15 ouncecan of cannellini beans
- Juice from 1 lemon
- 2 tablespoons fresh dill, chopped
- 5 fresh mint leaves
- ½ cup coconut milk
- Fresh herbs and peas, to garnish

Directions:
- In a slow cooker, add olive oil and onion.
- Sauté for 2 minutes then toss in the rest of the soup ingredients.
- Put on the slow cooker's lid and Cooking
- Time: for 2 hours on low heat.
- Once done, blend the soup with a hand blender.
- Garnish with fresh herbs and peas.
- Serve warm.

88) Swiss Coco Whisked Egg Soup

Preparation Time: 15 minutes

Cooking Time: 10 minutes

Servings: 4

Nutrition: Calories: 185 Carbs: 2.9g Fats: 11g Proteins: 18.3g

Ingredients:
- 3 cups bone broth
- 2 eggs, whisked
- 1 teaspoon ground oregano
- 3 tablespoons butter
- 2 cups Swiss chard, chopped
- 2 tablespoons coconut aminos
- 1 teaspoon ginger, grated
- Black pepper, to taste

Directions:
- Heat the bone broth in a saucepan and add whisked eggs while stirring slowly. Add the swiss chard, butter, coconut aminos, ginger, oregano and black pepper. Cook for about 10 minutes and serve hot.

89) Spinach and Mushroom Soup with Fresh Cream

Preparation Time: 15 minutes

Cooking Time: 10 minutes

Servings: 4

Nutrition: Calories: 160 Carbs: 7g Fats: 13.3g Proteins: 4.7g

Ingredients:
- 1 cup spinach, cleaned and chopped
- 100g mushrooms, chopped
- 1onion
- 6 garlic cloves
- ½ teaspoon red chili powder
- Black pepper, to taste
- 3 tablespoons buttermilk
- 1 teaspoon almond flour
- 2 cups chicken broth
- 3 tablespoons butter
- ¼ cup fresh cream for garnish

Directions:
- Heat butter in a pan and add onions and garlic. Sauté for about 3 minutes and add spinach and red chili powder.
- Sauté for about 4 minutes and add mushrooms. Transfer into a blender and blend to make a puree. Return to the pan and add buttermilk and almond flour for creamy texture.
- Mix well and simmer for about 2 minutes. Garnish with fresh cream and serve hot.

90) Veggie Soup with Peanut Butter

Preparation Time: 10 minutes

Cooking Time: 4 hrs. 5 minutes

Servings: 06

Nutrition: Calories 201 Fat 8.9 g Carbs 24.7 g Protein 15.3 g

Ingredients:
- 1 tablespoon water
- 6 cups sweet potatoes, peeled and chopped
- 2 cups onions, chopped
- 1 cup celery, chopped
- 4 large cloves garlic, chopped
- 2 teaspoons cumin seeds
- 3½ teaspoons ground coriander
- 1 teaspoon paprika
- ½ teaspoon crushed red pepper flakes
- 2 cups vegetable stock
- 3 cups water
- 4 tablespoons fresh ginger, grated
- 2 tablespoons natural peanut butter
- 2 cups cooked chickpeas
- 4 tablespoons lime juice
- Fresh cilantro, chopped
- Chopped peanuts, to garnish

Directions:
- In a slow cooker, add olive oil and onion.
- Sauté for 5 minutes then toss in the rest of the soup ingredients except chickpeas.
- Put on the slow cooker's lid and Cooking Time: for 4 hours on low heat.
- Once done, blend the soup with a hand blender.
- Stir in chickpeas and garnish with cilantro and peanuts.
- Serve warm.

91) Simple Red Lentil Soup

Preparation Time: 40 minutes

Cooking Time:

Servings: 3

Nutrition: Carbs: 15.3 g **Protein:** 6.2 g **Fats:** 0.3 g **Calories:** 90

Ingredients:
- Split red lentils: 1 cup
- Carrots: 1 cup grated
- Water: 6 cups
- Onion: 1 large coarsely chopped

Directions:
- Take a large saucepan and add water and bring to boil
- Add the chopped onions, carrots, lentils and bring to boil
- Lower the heat to medium and Cooking
- Time: for 20 minutes with partial cover
- Add the mixture to the high-speed blender to make a puree
- Whisk in water if desired
- Add again to the pan and slowly heat on a low flame for 10-15 minutes
- Add herbs or spices in between to augment the taste

92) Creamy Squash Soup

Preparation Time: 15 minutes

Cooking Time: 27 minutes

Servings: 5

Nutrition: Calories: 109 **Carbs:** 4.9g **Fats:** 8.5g **Proteins:** 3g

Ingredients:
- 1½ cups beef bone broth
- 1 small onion, peeled and grated.
- ¼ teaspoon poultry seasoning
- 2 small Delicata Squash, chopped
- 2 garlic cloves, minced
- 2 tablespoons olive oil
- ¼ teaspoon black pepper
- 1 small lemon, juiced
- 5 tablespoons sour cream

Directions:
- Put Delicata Squash and water in a medium pan and bring to a boil. Reduce the heat and cook for about 20 minutes. Drain and set aside.
- Put olive oil, onions, garlic and poultry seasoning in a small sauce pan. Cook for about 2 minutes and add broth. Allow it to simmer for 5 minutes and remove from heat.
- Whisk in the lemon juice and transfer the mixture in a blender. Pulse until smooth and top with sour cream.

93) Asparagus and Seed Soup with Cashew Cream

Preparation Time: 30 minutes

Cooking Time:

Servings: 2

Nutrition: Carbs: 11 g **Protein:** 9.4 g **Fats:** 18.3 g **Calories:** 243.5

Ingredients:
- Asparagus: 2 cups
- Vegetable stock: 4 cups
- Sesame seed: 2 tbsp
- Lemon juice: 1 tbsp
- Garlic: 4 cloves crushed
- Cashew cream: ½ cup
- Onion: 1 chopped
- Olive oil: 2 tbsp
- Pepper: as per your taste

Directions:
- Take a large saucepan and add olive oil to it
- Fry onion and garlic till it turns golden brown
- Chop asparagus and add to the pan along with the vegetable stock
- Let it boil and then Cooking Time: on low heat for 20 minutes
- When ready, add sesame seeds, lemon juice, and pepper as per your taste
- Serve with cashew cream on top

94) Spicy Bean Carrot and Lentil Soup

Preparation Time: 45 minutes

Cooking Time:

Servings: 4

Nutrition: Carbs: 425 g Protein: 8.17 g Fats: 4 g Calories: 148.75

Ingredients:
- Red lentils: 1 cup washed and drained
- Carrot: 2 medium chopped
- Beans: 1 cup drained
- Water: 3 cups
- Garlic: 3 cloves minced
- Onion: 1 medium finely chopped
- Ground cumin: 1 tsp
- Nutmeg: 1 tsp
- Ground coriander: 1 tsp
- Ground allspice: 1 tsp
- Ground cinnamon: 1 tsp
- Ground cayenne: ½ tsp
- Black pepper: as per your taste
- Extra virgin olive oil: 2 tbsp
- Cilantro: 1 tbsp chopped

Directions:
- Take a soup pot and heat oil in it on a medium flame
- Add onion and fry for 4-5 minutes
- Add carrot and garlic and stir for 5 minutes
- Wash lentils and add them to the pot
- Add water and bring to boil
- Lower the heat and Cooking Time: and cover for 15 minutes till lentil softens
- Add the remaining ingredients except for cilantro and Cooking Time: for an additional 15 minutes
- Serve warm with cilantro on top

95) Broccoli Ginger Soup with Herbs

Preparation Time: 15 minutes

Cooking Time: 37 minutes

Servings: 6

Nutrition: Calories: 183 Carbs: 5.2g Fats: 15.6g Proteins: 6.1g

Ingredients:
- 3 tablespoons ghee
- 5 garlic cloves
- 1 teaspoon sage
- ¼ teaspoon ginger
- 2 cups broccoli
- 1 small onion
- 1 teaspoon oregano
- ½ teaspoon parsley
- Black pepper, to taste
- 6 cups vegetable broth
- 4 tablespoons butter

Directions:
- Put ghee, onions, spices and garlic in a pot and cook for 3 minutes. Add broccoli and cook for about 4 minutes. Add vegetable broth, cover and allow it to simmer for about 30 minutes.
- Transfer into a blender and blend until smooth. Add the butter to give it a creamy delicious texture and flavor

96) Creamy Kabocha Soup

Preparation Time: 15 minutes

Cooking Time: 39 minutes

Servings: 8

Nutrition: Calories: 186 Carbs: 10.4g Fats: 14.9g Proteins: 3.7g

Ingredients:
- 1 apple, chopped
- 1 whole kabocha pumpkin, peeled, seeded and cubed
- 1 cup almond flour
- ¼ cup ghee
- 1 pinch cardamom powder
- 2 quarts water
- ¼ cup coconut cream
- 1 pinch ground black pepper

Directions:
- Heat ghee in the bottom of a heavy pot and add apples. Cook for about 5 minutes on a medium flame and add pumpkin.
- Sauté for about 3 minutes and add almond flour. Sauté for about 1 minute and add water. Lower the flame and cook for about 30 minutes.
- Transfer the soup into an immersion blender and blend until smooth. Top with coconut cream and serve.

97) Beans and Green Soup

Preparation Time: 20 minutes

Cooking Time:

Servings: 3

Nutrition: Carbs: 29.86 g Protein: 12.9 g Fats: 1.2 g Calories: 144

Ingredients:
- Cannellini beans: 1 cup rinsed and drained
- Artichoke hearts: 2 cups drained and chopped
- Frozen chopped spinach: 2 cups
- Water: 3 cups + 1 cup
- Garlic: 4 cloves chopped
- Onion: 1 medium chopped
- Italian herb blend: 2 tsp
- Black pepper: as per your taste

Directions:
- Take a blender and add onion, garlic, drained beans, herb blend, and pepper and add water
- Blend to give a smooth texture
- Add this puree to a large pan and Cooking Time: on medium-high heat
- When it initiates to boil, lower the heat and stir in between
- Let the mixture to thicken a bit
- Add one cup of water and spinach and blend
- Also, add artichokes and heat for 5 minutes
- Season with pepper if desired and serve

98) Sweety Onion Soup

Preparation Time: 15 minutes

Cooking Time: 335 minutes

Servings: 6

Nutrition: Calories: 198 Carbs: 6g Fats: 19.6g Proteins: 2.9g

Ingredients:
- 5 tablespoons butter
- 500 g brown onion medium
- 4 drops liquid stevia
- 4 tablespoons olive oil
- 3 cups beef stock

Directions:
- Put the butter and olive oil in a large pot over medium low heat and add onions. Cook for about 5 minutes and stir in stevia.
- Cook for another 5 minutes and add beef stock. Reduce the heat to low and simmer for about 25 minutes. Dish out into soup bowls and serve hot.

99) Lentils and Bean Mix in Masala Soup

Preparation Time: 40 minutes

Cooking Time:

Servings: 2

Nutrition: Carbs: 51.5 g Protein: 19.1 g Fats: 15.3 g Calories: 420

Ingredients:
- Red lentils: 1 cups
- Tomatoes: 1 cup can diced
- Beans: 1 cup can rinsed and drained
- Garam masala: 1 tbsp
- Vegetable oil: 2 tbsp
- Onion: 1 cup chopped
- Garlic: 3 cloves minced
- Ground cumin: 2 tbsp
- Smoked paprika: 1 tsp
- Celery: 1 cup chopped
- Lime juice and zest: 3 tbsp
- Fresh cilantro: 3 tbsp chopped
- Water: 2 cups

Directions:
- Take a large pot and add oil to it
- On the medium flame, add garlic, celery and onion
- Add garam masala, and cumin to them and stir for 5 minutes till they turn brown
- Add water, lentils, and tomatoes with the juice and bring to boil
- Bring to boil and heat for 25-30 minutes on low flame
- Add in lime juice and zest and beans of your choice and stir
- Serve with cilantro on top

100) Cauli Soup with Matcha Tea

Preparation Time: 15 minutes

Cooking Time: 13 minutes

Servings: 6

Nutrition: Calories: 79 Carbs: 3.8g Fats: 7.1g Proteins: 1.3g

Ingredients:
- 2 teaspoons thyme powder
- 1 head cauliflower
- 3 cups vegetable stock
- ½ teaspoon matcha green tea powder
- 3 tablespoons olive oil
- Black pepper, to taste
- 5 garlic cloves, chopped

Directions:
- Put the vegetable stock, thyme and matcha powder to a large pot over medium-high heat and bring to a boil. Add cauliflower and cook for about 10 minutes.
- Meanwhile, put the olive oil and garlic in a small sauce pan and cook for about 1 minute. Add the garlic and black pepper and cook for about 2 minutes.
- Transfer into an immersion blender and blend until smooth. Dish out and serve immediately.

Chapter 7 - Snack Recipe

101) Smoked Thaini Beets Hummus

Preparation Time: 10 minutes

Cooking Time: 60 minutes

Servings: 4

Nutrition: Calories: 50.1 Cal Fat: 2.5 g Carbs: 5 g Protein: 2 g

Ingredients:
- 15 ounces cooked chickpeas
- 3 small beets
- 1 teaspoon minced garlic
- 1/2 teaspoon smoked paprika
- 1/4 teaspoon red chili flakes
- 2 tablespoons olive oil
- 1 lemon, juiced
- 2 tablespoon tahini
- 1 tablespoon chopped almonds
- 1 tablespoon chopped cilantro

Directions:
- Drizzle oil over beets, then wrap beets in a foil and bake for 60 minutes at 425 degrees F until tender.
- When done, let beet cool for 10 minutes, then peel and dice them and place them in a food processor.
- Add remaining ingredients and pulse for 2 minutes until smooth, tip the hummus in a bowl, drizzle with some more oil, and then serve straight away.

102) Lemony Fava Cream

Preparation Time: 10 minutes

Cooking Time: 30 minutes

Servings: 4

Nutrition: Calories 405 Fat 1 g Carbs 75 g Protein 25 g

Ingredients:
- 2 cups Santorini fava (yellow split peas), rinsed
- 2 medium onions, chopped
- 2 ½ cups water
- 2 cups +2 tablespoons vegetable broth
- To garnish:
- Lemon juice as required
- Chopped parsley

Directions:
- Place fava in a large pot. Add onions, broth, water and stir. Place over medium heat. When it begins to boil, reduce the heat and cook until fava is tender.
- Remove from heat and cool. Blend until creamy. Ladle into small plates. Add lemon juice and stir. Garnish with parsley and serve.

103) Zucchini Hummus with Cumin

Preparation Time: 5 minutes

Cooking Time: 0 minute

Servings: 8

Nutrition: Calories: 65 Cal Fat: 5 g Carbs: 3 g Protein: 2 g

Ingredients:
- 1 cup diced zucchini
- 1 teaspoon minced garlic
- 2 teaspoons ground cumin
- 3 tablespoons lemon juice
- 1/3 cup tahini

Directions:
- Place all the ingredients in a food processor and pulse for 2 minutes until smooth.
- Tip the hummus in a bowl, drizzle with oil and serve.

104) Crispy Hummus Bell Pepper

Preparation Time: 10 minutes

Cooking Time: 0 minutes

Servings: 2

Nutrition: Calories 136 Fat 7 g Carbs 13 g Protein 6 g

Ingredients:
- 4 tablespoons hummus
- 2 large whole grain crisp bread
- 4 tablespoons crumbled feta
- 1 small bell pepper, diced

Directions:
- Top the pieces of crisp bread with hummus. Sprinkle feta cheese and bell peppers and serve.

105) Totopos Enchilados

Preparation Time: 10 minutes

Cooking Time: 15 minutes

Servings: 4

Nutrition: Calories: 150 Fat: 7 g Carbs: 18 g Protein: 2 g

Ingredients:
- 12 ounces whole-wheat tortillas
- 4 tablespoons chipotle seasoning
- 1 tablespoon olive oil
- 4 limes, juiced

Directions:
- Whisk together oil and lime juice, brush it well on tortillas, then sprinkle with chipotle seasoning and bake for 15 minutes at 350 degrees F until crispy, turning halfway.
- When done, let the tortilla cool for 10 minutes, then break it into chips and serve.

106) Garlic Tomato Italian Toast

Preparation Time: 10 minutes

Cooking Time: 10 minutes

Servings: 3

Nutrition: Calories 162 Fat 4 g Carbs 29 g Protein 4 g

Ingredients:
- 3 tomatoes, finely chopped
- 1 clove garlic, minced
- ¼ teaspoon garlic powder (optional)
- A handful basil leaves, coarsely chopped
- Pepper to taste
- ½ teaspoon olive oil
- ½ tablespoon balsamic vinegar
- ½ tablespoon butter
- ½ baguette French bread or Italian bread, cut into ½ inch thick slices

Directions:
- Add tomatoes, garlic and basil in a bowl and toss well. Add pepper. Drizzle oil and vinegar and toss well. Set aside for an hour.
- Melt the butter and brush it over the baguette slices. Place in an oven and toast the slices. Sprinkle the tomato mixture on top and serve right away.

107) Spanish Potato Tortillas

Preparation Time: 10 minutes

Cooking Time: 8 minutes

Servings: 10

Nutrition: Calories: 70 Fat: 3 g Carbs: 8 g Protein: 1 g

Ingredients:
- 1/3 cup quinoa flour
- 1½ cups shredded sweet potato
- 1 cup grated carrot
- 1/3 teaspoon ground black pepper
- 2 teaspoons curry powder
- 2 flax eggs
- 2 tablespoons coconut oil

Directions:
- Place all the ingredients in a bowl, except for oil, stir well until combined and then shape the mixture into ten small patties
- Take a large pan, place it over medium-high heat, add oil and when it melts, add patties in it and Cooking Time: for 3 minutes per side until browned.
- Serve straight away

108) Turkish Delicious Spiced Falafel

Preparation Time: 30 minutes

Cooking Time: 15 minutes

Servings: 2

Nutrition: Calories 93 Fat 3.8 g Carbs 1.3 g Protein 3.9 g

Ingredients:
- 1 cup dried chickpeas (do not use cooked or canned)
- ½ cup fresh parsley leaves, discard stems
- ¼ cup fresh dill leaves, discard stems
- ½ cup fresh cilantro leaves
- 4 cloves garlic, peeled
- ½ tablespoon ground black pepper
- ½ tablespoon ground coriander
- ½ tablespoon ground cumin
- ½ teaspoon cayenne pepper (optional)
- ½ teaspoon baking powder
- ¼ teaspoon baking soda
- 1 tablespoon toasted sesame seeds
- Oil, as required

Directions:
- Rinse chickpeas and soak in water overnight. Cover with at least 3 inches of water. Drain and dry by patting with a kitchen towel.
- Add all the fresh herbs into a food processor. Process until finely chopped. Add chickpeas, spices and garlic and pulse for not more than 40 seconds each time until smooth.
- Transfer into a container. Cover and chill for at least 1 hour or until use. Divide the mixture into 12 equal portions and shape into patties.
- Place a deep pan over medium heat. Pour enough oil to cover at least 3 inches from the bottom of the pan.
- When the oil is well heated, but not smoking, drop falafel, a few at a time and fry until medium brown.
- Remove with a spoon and place on a plate lined with paper towels. Serve with a dip of your choice.

109) Red Pesto Bruschetta

Preparation Time: 5 minutes

Cooking Time: 0 minute

Servings: 4

Nutrition: Calories: 214 Fat: 7.2 g Carbs: 32 g Protein: 6.5 g

Ingredients:
- 1 small tomato, sliced
- ¼ teaspoon ground black pepper
- 1 tablespoon vegan pesto
- 2 tablespoons hummus
- 1 slice of whole-grain bread, toasted
- Hemp seeds as needed for garnishing

Directions:
- Spread hummus on one side of the toast, top with tomato slices and then drizzle with pesto.
- Sprinkle black pepper on the toast along with hemp seeds and then serve straight away.

110) Cheesy Low-Fat Yogurt Dip

Preparation Time: 15 minutes + chilling

Cooking Time: 0 minutes

Servings: 8 (2 tablespoons dip without vegetable sticks)

Nutrition: Calories 68 Fat 4 g Carbs 5 g Protein 4 g

Ingredients:
- 2 cups plain low-fat yogurt
- ¼ cup crumbled feta cheese
- 3 tablespoons chopped walnuts or pine nuts
- 1 teaspoon chopped fresh oregano or marjoram or ½ teaspoon dried oregano or marjoram, crushed
- Freshly ground pepper to taste
- 1 tablespoon snipped dried tomatoes (not oil packed)
- Walnut halves to garnish
- Assorted vegetable sticks to serve

Directions:
- For yogurt dip, place 3 layers of cotton cheesecloth over a strainer. Place strainer over a bowl. Add yogurt into the strainer. Cover the strainer with cling wrap. Refrigerate for 24-48 hours.
- Discard the strained liquid and add yogurt into a bowl. Add feta cheese, walnuts, seasoning, and herbs and mix well. Cover and chill for an hour.
- Garnish with walnut halves. Serve with vegetable sticks.

111) Exotic Hummus And Sprout Toast

Preparation Time: 5 minutes

Cooking Time: 0 minute

Servings: 4

Nutrition: Calories: 200 Fat: 10.5 g Carbs: 22 g Protein: 7 g

Ingredients:
- 1/2 of a medium avocado, sliced
- 1 slice of whole-grain bread, toasted
- 2 tablespoons sprouts
- 2 tablespoons hummus
- ¼ teaspoon lemon zest
- ½ teaspoon hemp seeds
- ¼ teaspoon red pepper flakes

Directions:
- Spread hummus on one side of the toast and then top with avocado slices and sprouts.
- Sprinkle with lemon zest, hemp seeds, and red pepper flakes and then serve straight away.

112) Rich Ricotta Snack

Preparation Time: 5 minutes

Cooking Time: 0 minutes

Servings: 2

Nutrition: Calories 178 Fat 9 g Carbs 15 g Protein 11 g

Ingredients:
- 2/3 cup part-skim ricotta
- 2 clementine's, peeled, separated into segments, deseeded
- 4 teaspoons chopped pistachio nuts

Directions:
- Place 1/3 cup ricotta in each of 2 bowls. Divide the clementine segments equally and place over the ricotta. Sprinkle pistachio nuts on top and serve.

113) Sweety Apple Toast with Cinnamon

Preparation Time: 5 minutes

Cooking Time: 0 minute

Servings: 4

Nutrition: Calories: 212 Fat: 7 g Carbs: 35 g Protein: 4 g

Ingredients:
- ½ of a small apple, cored, sliced
- 1 slice of whole-grain bread, toasted
- 1 tablespoon honey
- 2 tablespoons hummus
- 1/8 teaspoon cinnamon

Directions:
- Spread hummus on one side of the toast, top with apple slices and then drizzle with honey.
- Sprinkle cinnamon on it and then serve straight away.

114) Crispy Zucchini

Preparation Time: 10 minutes

Cooking Time: 120 minutes

Servings: 4

Nutrition: Calories: 54 Fat: 5 g Carbs: 1 g Protein: 6 g

Ingredients:
- 1 large zucchini, thinly sliced
- 2 tablespoons olive oil

Directions:
- Pat dry zucchini slices and then spread them in an even layer on a baking sheet lined with parchment sheet.
- Add oil, brush this mixture over zucchini slices on both sides and then bake for 2 hours or more until brown and crispy.
- When done, let the chips cool for 10 minutes and then serve straight away.

115) Summer Vegetarian Wraps

Preparation Time: 15 minutes

Cooking Time: 10 minutes

Servings: 2

Nutrition: Calories: 262; Fat: 15g; Carbs: 23g; Protein: 7g

Ingredients:
- 1½ cups seedless cucumber, peeled and chopped (about 1 large cucumber)
- 1 cup chopped tomato (about 1 large tomato)
- ½ cup finely chopped fresh mint
- 1 (2.25-ounce) can sliced black olives (about ½ cup), drained
- ¼ cup diced red onion (about ¼ onion)
- 2 tablespoons extra-virgin olive oil
- 1 tablespoon red wine vinegar
- ¼ teaspoon freshly ground black pepper
- ½ cup crumbled goat cheese (about 2 ounces)
- 4 whole-wheat flatbread wraps or soft whole-wheat tortillas

Directions:
- In a large bowl, mix together the cucumber, tomato, mint, olives, and onion until well combined.
- In a small bowl, whisk together the oil, vinegar, and pepper. Drizzle the dressing over the salad, and mix gently.
- With a knife, spread the goat cheese evenly over the four wraps. Spoon a quarter of the salad filling down the middle of each wrap.
- Fold up each wrap: Start by folding up the bottom, then fold one side over and fold the other side over the top. Repeat with the remaining wraps and serve.

116) Spiced Pineapple Mix

Preparation Time: 15 minutes

Cooking Time: 90 minutes

Servings: 4

Nutrition: Calories: 230 Fat: 17.5 g Carbs: 11.5 g Protein: 6.5 g

Ingredients:
- 5 cups mixed nuts
- 1 cup chopped dried pineapple
- 1 cup pumpkin seed
- 1 teaspoon garlic powder
- 1 teaspoon onion powder
- 2 teaspoons paprika
- 1/4 cup coconut sugar
- 1/2 teaspoon red chili powder
- 1/2 teaspoon ground black pepper
- 1 tablespoon red pepper flakes
- 1/2 tablespoon red curry powder
- 2 tablespoons soy sauce
- 2 tablespoons coconut oil

Directions:
- Switch on the slow cooker, add all the ingredients in it except for dried pineapple and red pepper flakes, stir until combined and Cooking Time: for 90 minutes at high heat setting, stirring every 30 minutes.
- When done, spread the nut mixture on a baking sheet lined with parchment paper and let it cool.
- Then spread dried pineapple on top, sprinkle with red pepper flakes and serve.

117) Salmon Wraps with Balsamic Vinegar

Preparation Time: 20 minutes

Cooking Time: 60 minutes

Servings: 2

Nutrition: Calories: 336; Total Fat: 16g; Carbs: 23g; Protein: 32g

Ingredients:
- 1-pound salmon filet, cooked and flaked, or 3 (5-ounce) cans salmon
- ½ cup diced carrots (about 1 carrot)
- ½ cup diced celery (about 1 celery stalk)
- 3 tablespoons chopped fresh dill
- 3 tablespoons diced red onion (a little less than 1/8 onion)
- 2 tablespoons capers
- 1½ tablespoons extra-virgin olive oil
- 1 tablespoon aged balsamic vinegar
- ½ teaspoon freshly ground black pepper
- 4 whole-wheat flatbread wraps or soft whole-wheat tortillas

Directions:
- In a large bowl, mix together the salmon, carrots, celery, dill, red onion, capers, oil, vinegar and pepper.
- Divide the salmon salad among the flatbreads. Fold up the bottom of the flatbread, then roll up the wrap and serve.

118) Incredible Dried Snack

Preparation Time: 10 minutes

Cooking Time: 17 minutes

Servings: 2

Nutrition: 44g Carbs, 7g Fat, 13g Protein, 285 Calories 65

Ingredients:
- 3 c. water
- ¼ c. cashew nut
- 8 dried apricots
- 4 dried figs
- 1 tsp. cinnamon

Directions:
- In a pot, mix water and quinoa and
- Let simmer for 15 minutes, until the water evaporates.
- Chop dried fruit.
- When quinoa is cooked, stir in all other ingredients.
- Serve cold. Add milk, if desired.

119) *Crispy Beet with Rosemary*

Preparation Time: 10 minutes

Cooking Time: 20 minutes

Servings: 3

Nutrition: Calories: 79 Fat: 4.7 g Carbs: 8.6 g Protein: 1.5 g

Ingredients:
- 3 large beets, scrubbed, thinly sliced
- 1/8 teaspoon ground black pepper
- 3 sprigs of rosemary, leaves chopped
- 4 tablespoons olive oil

Directions:
- Spread beet slices in a single layer between two large baking sheets, brush the slices with oil, then season with spices and rosemary, toss until well coated, and bake for 20 minutes at 375 degrees F until crispy, turning halfway.
- When done, let the chips cool for 10 minutes and then serve.

120) *Sweety Oats with Cinnamon*

Preparation Time: 10 minutes

Cooking Time: 15 minutes

Servings: 2

Nutrition: Calories: 232, Fat: 5.7 g, Carbs: 48.1 g, Protein: 5.2 g

Ingredients:
- ½ tsp. cinnamon
- ¼ tsp. ginger
- 2 apples make half-inch chunks
- ½ c. oats, steel cut
- 1½ c. water
- Maple syrup
- Clove
- ¼ tsp. nutmeg

Directions:
- Take Instant Pot and careful y arrange it over a clean, dry kitchen platform.
- Turn on the appliance.
- In the cooking pot area, add the water, oats, cinnamon, ginger, clove, nutmeg and apple. Stir the ingredients gently.
- Close the pot lid and seal the valve to avoid any leakage. Find and press the "Manual" cooking setting and set cooking time to 5 minutes.
- Allow the recipe ingredients to cook for the set time, and after that, the timer reads "zero."
- Press "Cancel" and press "NPR" setting for natural pressure release. It takes 8-10 times for all inside pressure to release.
- Open the pot and arrange the cooked recipe in serving plates.
- Sweeten as needed with maple or agave syrup and serve immediately.
- Top with some chopped nuts, optional.

Chapter 8 -   Dessert and Smoothie Recipes

121) Cocoflakes Cantaloupe Yogurt with Raspberry

Preparation Time: 15 minutes

Cooking Time: 0 minutes

Servings: 6

Nutrition: Calories: 75 Fat: 4.1g Protein: 1.2g Carbs: 10.9g

Ingredients:
- 2 cups fresh raspberries, mashed
- 1 cup plain coconut yogurt
- ½ teaspoon vanilla extract
- 1 cantaloupe, peeled and sliced
- ½ cup toasted coconut flakes

Directions:
- Combine the mashed raspberries with yogurt and vanilla extract in a small bowl. Stir to mix well.
- Place the cantaloupe slices on a platter, then top with raspberry mixture and spread with toasted coconut. Serve immediately.

122) Plant-Based Berry and Banana Smoothie

Preparation Time: 5 minutes

Cooking Time:

Servings: 2

Nutrition: Calories 269, Fat 12.3g, Carbs 37.6g, Protein 6.4g

Ingredients:
- 2 cups, plant-based Milk
- 2 cups, Frozen or fresh berries
- ½ cup Frozen ripe bananas
- 2 teaspoons, Flax Seeds
- ¼ tsp, Vanilla
- ¼ tsp, Cinnamon

Directions:
- Mix together milk, flax seeds, and fruit. Blend in a high-power blender.
- Add cinnamon and vanilla. Blend until smooth.
- Serve and enjoy!

123) Delicious Apple Compote with Cinnamon

Preparation Time: 15 minutes

Cooking Time: 10 minutes

Servings: 4

Nutrition: Calories: 246 Fat: 0.9g Protein: 1.2g Carbs: 66.3g

Ingredients:
- 6 apples, peeled, cored, and chopped
- ¼ cup raw honey
- 1 teaspoon ground cinnamon
- ¼ cup apple juice

Directions:
- Put all the ingredients in a stockpot. Stir to mix well, then cook over medium-high heat for 10 minutes or until the apples are glazed by honey and lightly saucy. Stir constantly. Serve immediately.

124) Carrot and Prunes Smoothie with Walnuts

Preparation Time: 5 minutes

Cooking Time:

Servings: 4

Nutrition: Carbs: 14.9 g Protein: 3 g Fats: 4.5 g Calories: 103

Ingredients:
- Almond milk: 2 cups
- Prunes: 60 g
- Banana: 1
- Carrots: 150 g
- Walnuts: 30 g
- Ground cinnamon: ½ tsp
- Vanilla extract: 1 tsp

Directions:
- Add all the ingredients to the blender
- Blend on high speed to make it smooth

125) Choco Bombs

Preparation Time: 45 minutes

Cooking Time: 0 minutes

Servings: 15 balls

Nutrition: Calories: 146 Fat: 8.1g Protein: 4.2g Carbs: 16.9g

Ingredients:
- ¾ cup creamy peanut butter
- ¼ cup unsweetened cocoa powder
- 2 tablespoons softened almond butter
- ½ teaspoon vanilla extract
- 1¾ cups maple sugar

Directions:
- Line a baking sheet with parchment paper. Combine all the ingredients in a bowl. Stir to mix well.
- Divide the mixture into 15 parts and shape each part into a 1-inch ball. Arrange the balls on the baking sheet and refrigerate for at least 30 minutes, then serve chilled.

126) Dark Date and Banana Drink

Preparation Time: 5 minutes

Cooking Time:

Servings: 2

Nutrition: Carbs: 72.1 g Protein: 8 g Fats: 12.7 g Calories: 385

Ingredients:
- Unsweetened cocoa powder: 2 tbsp
- Unsweetened nut milk: 2 cups
- Almond butter: 2 tbsp
- Dried dates: 4 pitted
- Frozen bananas: 2 medium
- Ground cinnamon: ¼ tsp

Directions:
- Add all the ingredients to the blender
- Blend to form a smooth consistency

127) Sweety Watermelon Iced Flakes

Preparation Time: 10 minutes + 3 hours to freeze

Cooking Time: 0 minutes

Servings: 4

Nutrition: Calories: 153 **Carbs:** 39g **Protein:** 2g **Fat:** 1g

Ingredients:
- 4 cups watermelon cubes
- ¼ cup honey
- ¼ cup freshly squeezed lemon juice

Directions:
- In a blender, combine the watermelon, honey, and lemon juice. Purée all the ingredients, then pour into a 9-by-9-by-2-inch baking pan and place in the freezer.
- Every 30 to 60 minutes, run a fork across the frozen surface to fluff and create ice flakes. Freeze for about 3 hours total and serve.

128) Cashew and Fruit Mix Smoothie

Preparation Time: 5 minutes

Cooking Time:

Servings: 4

Nutrition: Carbs: 32.9 g **Protein:** 9.7 g **Fats:** 15 g **Calories:** 320

Ingredients:
- Pistachios: 1 cup
- Raw pumpkin: 175 g
- Cloves: 1
- Nutmeg: 1/8 tsp
- Dates: 4
- Banana: 1
- Ground ginger: 1/8 tsp
- Ground cinnamon: 1 tsp
- Cashew milk: 500 ml
- Ice: as per your need

Directions:
- Add all the ingredients to the blender
- Blend on high speed to make it smooth

129) Seed Butter Cookies

Preparation Time: 10 minutes

Cooking Time: 15 minutes

Servings: 14-16

Nutrition: Calories 218 **Fat** 12g **Carbs** 25g **Protein** 4g

Ingredients:
- 1 cup sesame seeds, hulled
- 1 cup sugar
- 8 tablespoons unsalted butter, softened
- 2 large eggs
- 1¼ cups flour

Directions:
- Preheat the oven to 350°F. Toast the sesame seeds on a baking sheet for 3 minutes. Set aside and let cool.
- Using a mixer, cream together the sugar and butter. Put the eggs one at a time until well-blended. Add the flour and toasted sesame seeds and mix until well-blended.
- Drop spoonful of cookie dough onto a baking sheet and form them into round balls, about 1-inch in diameter, similar to a walnut.
- Put in the oven and bake for 5 to 7 minutes or until golden brown. Let the cookies cool and enjoy.

130) Persimmon Healthy Smoothie

Preparation Time: 5 minutes

Cooking Time:

Servings: 1

Nutrition: Carbs: 37.1 g **Protein:** 6.5 g **Fats:** 5.4 g **Calories:** 183

Ingredients:
- Persimmon: 1
- Spinach: 1 cup
- Orange: 1
- Water: 1 cup
- Chia seeds: 1 tbsp

Directions:
- Add all the ingredients to the blender
- Blend to form a smooth consistency
- Add ice cubes from the top to chill it

131) Sweety Rice with Rose Water and Dried Figs

Preparation Time: 45 minutes

Cooking Time: 0 minutes

Servings: 2

Nutrition: Calories: 228; **Fat:** 6.1g; **Carbs:** 35.1g; **Protein:** 7.1g

Ingredients:
- 3 cups milk
- 1 cup water
- 2 tablespoons sugar
- 1/3 cup white rice, rinsed
- 1 tablespoon honey
- 4 dried figs, chopped
- 1/2 teaspoon cinnamon
- 1/2 teaspoon rose water

Directions:
- In a deep saucepan, bring the milk, water and sugar to a boil until the sugar has dissolved.
- Stir in the rice, honey, figs, raisins, cinnamon, and turn the heat to a simmer; let it simmer for about 40 minutes, stirring periodically to prevent your pudding from sticking.
- Afterwards, stir in the rose water. Divide the pudding between individual bowls and serve. Bon appétit!

132) Fresh and Dry Smoothie

Preparation Time: 5 minutes

Cooking Time:

Servings: 1

Nutrition: Carbs: 66.0 g Protein: 16.1 g Fats: 18 g Calories: 435

Ingredients:
- Fresh figs: 2
- Almond milk: 1 cup
- Dried date: 1 pitted
- Vanilla extract: ¼ tsp
- Sesame seeds: 2 tbsp

Directions:
- Add all the ingredients to the blender
- Blend to form a smooth consistency

133) Greek Yogurt with Honey and Fruit Mix

Preparation Time: 10 minutes

Cooking Time: 0 minutes

Servings: 2

Nutrition: Calories: 98; Fat: 0.2g; Carbs: 20.7g; Protein: 2.8g

Ingredients:
- 8 clementine orange segments
- 8 medium-sized strawberries
- 8 pineapple cubes
- 8 seedless grapes
- 1/2 cup Greek-style yogurt
- 1/2 teaspoon vanilla extract
- 2 tablespoons honey

Directions:
- Thread the fruits onto 4 skewers.
- In a mixing dish, thoroughly combine the yogurt, vanilla, and honey.
- Serve alongside your fruit kabobs for dipping. Bon appétit!

134) Almond Berries and Banana Smoothie

Preparation Time: 5 minutes

Cooking Time:

Servings: 2

Nutrition: Carbs: 14.9 g Protein: 2.2 g Fats: 1.6 g Calories: 92

Ingredients:
- Banana: 1 ripe
- Frozen berries: 200g
- Almond milk: 250ml

Directions:
- Add all the ingredients in the blender
- Blend to give a smooth consistency
- Pour to the glasses and serve

135) Choco Walnuts Cube with Thaini

Preparation Time: 10 minutes

Cooking Time: 0 minutes

Servings: 2

Nutrition: Calories: 198; Fat: 13g; Carbs: 17.3g; Protein: 4.6g

Ingredients:
- 8 ounces bittersweet chocolate
- 1 cup tahini paste
- 1/4 cup almonds, chopped
- 1/4 cup walnuts, chopped

Directions:
- Microwave the chocolate for about 30 seconds or until melted. Stir in the tahini, almonds, and walnuts.
- Spread the batter into a parchment-lined baking pan. Place in your refrigerator until set, for about 3 hours.
- Cut into cubes and serve well-chilled.

136) Fruit Explosion Smoothie

Preparation Time: 5 minutes

Cooking Time:

Servings: 2

Nutrition: Carbs: 52.8 g Protein: 6.4 g Fats: 19.5 g Calories: 407

Ingredients:
- Banana: 1 ripe sliced
- Almond milk: 1 cup
- Coconut oil: 1 tbsp
- Powdered ginger: 1 tsp
- Frozen fruit medley: 1 cup
- Chia seeds: 2 tbsp

Directions:
- Add all the ingredients in the blender
- Blend to give a smooth consistency
- Pour to the glasses and serve

137) Greek Granola Berries

Preparation Time: 10 minutes

Cooking Time: 0 minutes

Servings: 2

Nutrition: Calories: 238; Fat: 16.7g; Carbs: 53g; Protein: 21.6g

Ingredients:
- 2 cups Greek yogurt
- 2 cups mixed berries
- 1/2 cup granola

Directions:
- Alternate layers of mixed berries, granola, and yogurt until two dessert bowls are filled completely.
- Cover and place in your refrigerator until you're ready to serve. Bon appétit!

138) Energy Almond Smoothie

Preparation Time: 5 minutes

Cooking Time:

Servings: 1

Nutrition: Carbs: 41.2 g Protein: 8.9 g Fats: 3.9 g Calories: 220

Ingredients:
- Large banana: 1 frozen
- Fresh spinach: 1 cup
- Rolled oats: 2 tbsp
- Unsweetened almond milk: ¾ cup

Directions:
- Add all the ingredients to the blender
- Blend to form a smooth consistency

139) Figs and Walnuts with Honey Topping

Preparation Time: 20 Minutes

Cooking Time: 0 Minutes

Servings: 4

Nutrition: Calories: 110 Carbs: 26 Fat: 3g, Protein: 1g

Ingredients:
- 12 dried figs
- 2 Tbsps. thyme honey
- 2 Tbsps. sesame seeds
- 24 walnut halves

Directions:
- Cut off the tough stalk ends of the figs.
- Slice open each fig.
- Stuff the fig openings with two walnut halves and close
- Arrange the figs on a plate, drizzle with honey, and sprinkle the sesame seeds on it.
- Serve.

140) Thaini Figs Smoothie

Preparation Time: 5 minutes

Cooking Time:

Servings: 1

Nutrition: Carbs: 66.0 g

Protein: 12.1 g Fats: 16.5g Calories: 435

Ingredients:
- Dried date: 1 pitted
- Tahini: 1 tbsp
- Fresh figs: 2
- Almond milk: 1 cup
- Vanilla extract: ¼ tsp

Directions:
- Add all the ingredients to the blender
- Blend to form a smooth consistency

Chapter 9 - Simple Dr. Cole's Meal Plan – For Women

Day 1

3) Golden Coco Mix | Calories 259

21) Pasta with Delicious Spanish Salsa | Calories 364

62) Smoked Baby Spinach Stew | Calories 369

41) Veggie ChimiSalad | Calories 231

123) Delicious Apple Compote with Cinnamon | Calories 246

Total Calories: 1469

Day 2

10) Black Olives and Feta Bread | Calories 251

25) Chickpeas Tomato Pasta with Tamari | Calories 442

65) Veggie Ragù Noodles | Calories 353

46) Easy Creamy Kernel | Calories 306

125) Choco Bombs | Calories 146

Total Calories: 1498

Day 3

13) Vegetables Wraps with Soy Sauce | Calories 284

29) Spiced Kidney Pasta with Cilantro | Calories 274

67) Red Quinoa Burgers with Thaini Guacamole | Calories 343

48) Old School Panzanella | Calories 294

128) Cashew and Fruit Mix Smoothie | Calories 320

Total Calories: 1515

Day 4

19) Awesome Breakfast Muesli | Calories 250

31 Red Lentils Spaghetti with Herbs | Calories 335

72) Cold Spinach with Fruit Mix | Calories 296

53) Double Green Juicy Salad | Calories 237

140) Thaini Figs Smoothie | Calories 435

Total Calories: 1553

Day 5

7) Button Mushroom Omelette | Calories 189

35) Macaroni with Cherry and Peas | Calories 320

76) Hummus Quinoa with Edamame Bowl | Calories 381

56) Cheesy Asparagus Pesto Salad | Calories 220

138) Energy Almond Smoothie | Calories 220

Total Calories: 1330

Day 6

4) Delicious Agave Rice | Calories 192

37) Golden Rice with Pistachios | Calories 320

75) Cheesy Gnocchi with Shrimp | Calories 227

55) Asian Goji Salad | Calories 203

136) Fruit Explosion Smoothie | Calories 407

Total Calories: 1349

Day 7

2) Apple Warm Oatmeal | Calories 200

40) Bean Balls with Red pepper and Marinara Sauce | Calories 351

63) Green Chilis Chicken Breast | Calories 237

44) Noodles Salad with Peanut Butter Cream | Calories 361

126) Dark Date and Banana Drink | Calories 385

Total Calories: 1534

Chapter 10 - Conclusion

I hope this book of recipes will be useful to you in the long term, I remind you that the DASH diet is a diet proven by specialists from various medical disciplines, it is not just a fad or for aesthetic reasons, it will really make a difference in your life and your health.

The best medicine for our body is to take care of our diet, and if in addition to taking care of our health we can show off a better figure is the perfect deal.

Keep in mind that the portions that I include in each recipe must be careful so that the diet works properly and you get the most out of all the benefits it offers.

As a final tip, I suggest you write in your diary or in a notebook a note about how you feel before starting the diet, how you see your body, write down your weight, if you feel swollen or if you have heaviness, have any difficulty, in short your feelings in general, keep your notes and when you have at least two or three weeks of following this diet review it again and you will discover the changes that are already beginning to occur.

Much success and welcome to a healthier and happier life.

Lightning Source UK Ltd.
Milton Keynes UK
UKHW050237290521
384511UK00011B/595